AgelessBeauty

The secrets of aging beautifully

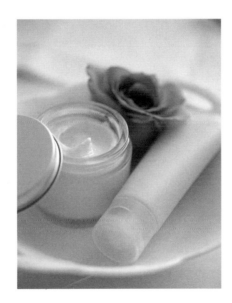

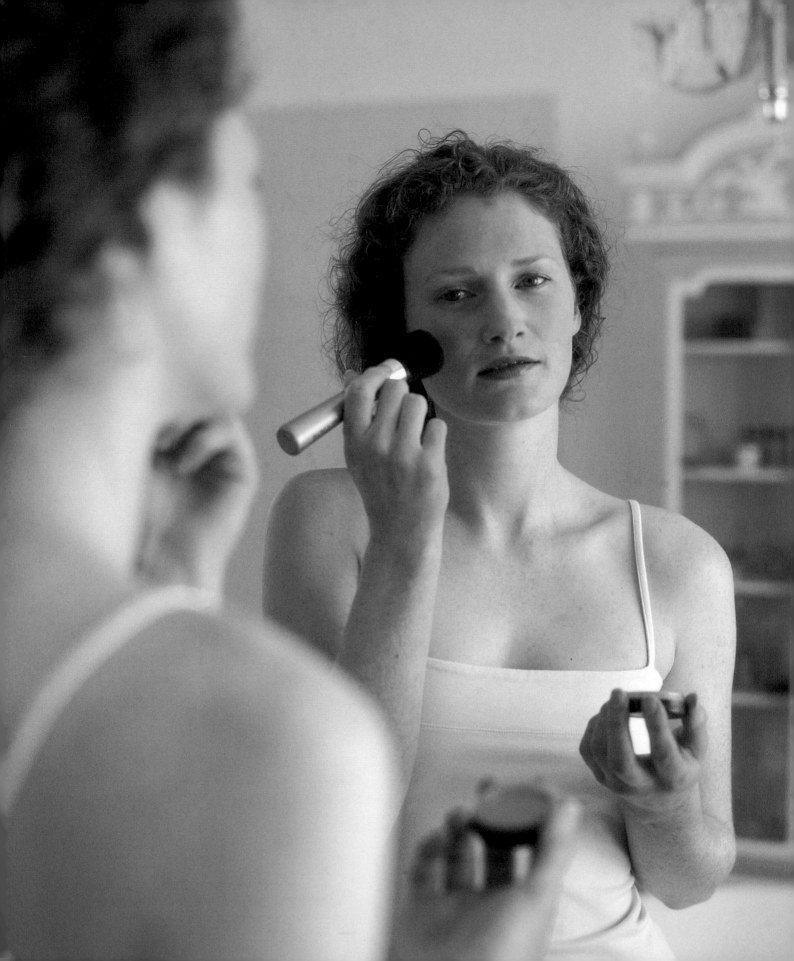

AgelessBeauty

The secrets of aging beautifully

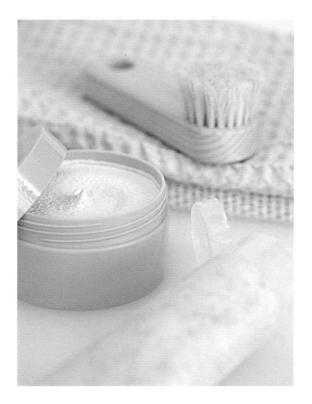

Liz Wilde

photography by Winfried Heinze

RYLAND
PETERS
& SMALL

LONDON NEW YORK

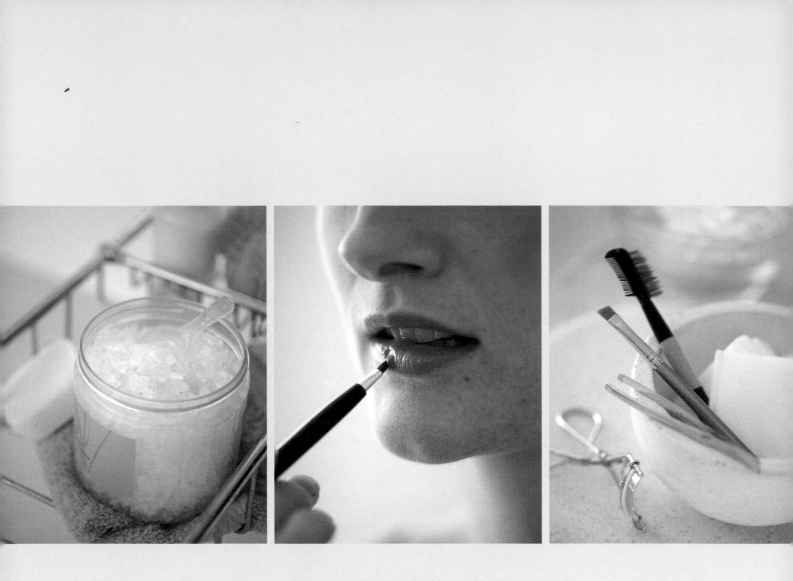

SENIOR DESIGNER Megan Smith
SENIOR EDITOR Clare Double
LOCATION RESEARCH Tracy Ogino
PRODUCTION Sheila Smith
ART DIRECTOR Anne-Marie Bulat
PUBLISHING DIRECTOR Alison Starling

STYLIST Liz Belton

First published in the United States in 2006
by Ryland Peters & Small
519 Broadway, 5th Floor
New York, NY 10012
www.rylandpeters.com

10 9 8 7 6 5 4 3 2 1

Library of Congress Cataloging-in-Publication Data

Wilde, Liz.
  Ageless beauty : the secrets of aging beautifully /
Liz Wilde ; photography by Winfried Heinze.
    p. cm.
  Includes index.
  ISBN-13: 978-1-84597-268-4
  ISBN-10: 1-84597-268-6
  1. Beauty, Personal. 2. Aging. I. Title.

RA778.W535 2006
646.7'042--dc22

                              2006011957

**To my wonderful mother,
who taught me that age
didn't matter.**

Contents

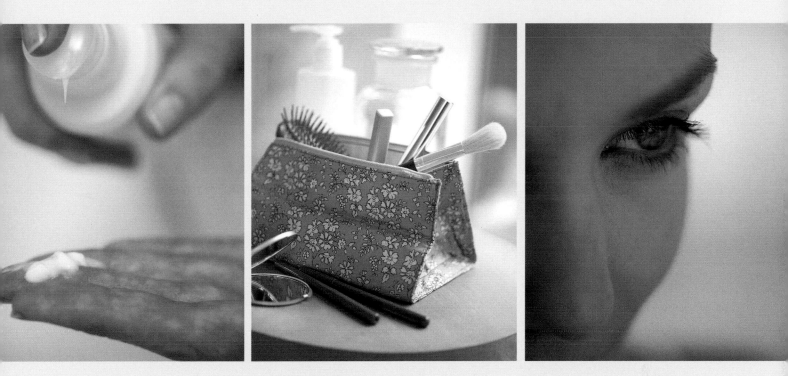

Introduction

As a society we've become obsessed with looking young, yet the images we're bombarded with every day are totally unrealistic. Cosmetic companies use teenage models to advertise their anti-aging creams, and "mature" Hollywood stars (i.e., anyone over 30) head straight for the Botox doctor or risk losing work. While studies have found that taking pride in your appearance makes you live longer, you will be pleased to know that this book is not simply about spending a fortune on face creams or painful injections. It's about the cheap (and often free) things you can do every day that make a massive difference to how good you look as you age.

First the facts. Some aspects of aging are unavoidable, such as your metabolic rate dropping a little each year, and gray hairs appearing. But the slippery slope of what most of us expect aging to be is optional. You don't need to put on weight. You don't need to get premature wrinkles. And you certainly don't need to suffer chronic aches and pains. Experts now believe an amazing 70% of what we feel as aging is optional. Plus, 80% of wrinkles are caused by environmental factors such as sun exposure and smoking, which means you can stop them developing. And the stuff you can't change—those gray hairs, for instance? We asked the experts—from makeup artists to hairdressers to skin specialists—for tricks on how to reverse (or hide) them.

Whatever your age or budget, this book contains hundreds of ways to help you look and feel younger for longer. You'll discover the major causes of aging and how to ensure they don't happen to you. You'll also find out how easy it is not to get old the way you think you have to. From eating an anti-aging diet to the proven power of your mind to delay (and even reverse) the aging process, this book will help you step off that slippery slope.

Within 15 years, one in five people in the West will be over 65. If you start making lifestyle changes now, you can look forward to a happy, healthy old age. New research says that over 50% of all illness and injury in the last third of your life can be prevented by changing your lifestyle. And most of what we associate with aging—aches and pains, low energy,

joint problems—can be put off for many, many years. The choice is yours. The more you look after your body, the more your body will look after you. This book isn't going to tell you to avoid life's pleasures and exist on mung beans for the rest of your days. But if you decide to stick with your sunbed and 20-a-day cigarette habit, don't be surprised if you look 50 when your birthday cards say 35. The truth is, you can choose to look and live young until you're well into old age by living consciously, and it's the little things you do every day that will make all the difference.

There was a time when 40 was middle-aged, but today we call it "middle youth." Years ago there was little we could do about aging. More recently we believed that a perma-tan was the perfect way to hide signs of aging. Little did we know how our skin would suffer for it later. Fortunately our health and beauty knowledge has improved significantly in the last few years, and we now know not only what ages us fast but also what simple things can make a real difference to how good we look and feel at any age. Remember, prevention is always easier than cure, which means it's no good investing in an expensive anti-wrinkle cream if you're going to spend your days stressed out in the office, or stretched out in the sun.

So, forget about growing old gracefully and instead decide to grow old brilliantly. You may not be able to change what it says on your birth certificate, but you can definitely slow down the rate your cells age. What goes into your body matters just as much as what goes onto your skin, hair, and nails. And, long term, what goes into your mind matters most of all. Recent research has found that optimists live 10 years longer than pessimists, with one 100-year-old lady saying she tried to make part of each day joyful rather than finding fault. So drop any anxieties about growing older and discover how to rejuvenate yourself inside and out. Hopefully this book will inspire you to take over the controls of how you age. The good news is simple. It's less about your genes than how you take care of yourself, which means you really can choose to live a significantly happier, healthier, and younger-looking life for longer than any generation before.

Age is opportunity no less
Than youth itself, though in
another dress.

LONGFELLOW

What's your Biological Age?

Forget what it says on your passport. The only age that really matters is your biological age—how old your body is in terms of wear and tear. This is measured by biomarkers such as memory, reaction, hearing, vision, agility, decision speed, movement speed, tactile sense, and lung function. Below are simple tests you can do at home, but for a detailed analysis take an inner age test (see Directory). Knowing if your body is older than its calendar years means you can take action to remedy and reverse the decline with simple lifestyle changes. The message is simple: much of your health is in your control.

Skin-fold thickness

Why? Being overweight increases your inner age, as it can put strain on other organs in your body.

The test: Hold your bare arm out horizontally with your forearm pointing vertically upward. Grasp the skin fold underneath your upper arm with your thumb and index finger, halfway between your armpit and elbow. Make sure the skin fold is the same length each side and avoid pinching the muscle. Ask a friend to measure the distance between your thumb and index finger.

1 in (2.5 cm) or less—6 points
All other results—2 points

Waist to hip ratio

Why? People with apple-shaped bodies (who carry excess weight around the waist) face more health risks than those who carry weight on their hips.

The test: Measure around your hips at the widest part of your bottom, and then measure the smallest part of your waist, usually just above the belly button. To get the ratio, divide your waist measurement by your hip measurement.

0.8 or less—6 points
All other results—2 points

Reaction

Why? Your reactions start to slow down in your 30s due to deterioration of tissue in the nerve fibers.

The test: Ask someone to hold a long ruler (at least 18 in, 45 cm) vertically above your dominant hand (i.e., right if you're right-handed) with the 1-inch mark end at the bottom. Ask them to let go and then try and catch the ruler as it drops. Make a note of where on the ruler you manage to grab.

6 in (15 cm) or less—8 points
6½–10 in (16–25 cm)—6 points
10½–12 in (26–30 cm)—4 points
12½–14 in (31–35 cm)—3 points
14½ in (36 cm) or more—2 points
You drop the ruler—0 points

Skin elasticity

Why? Sebum production declines as you age, making skin less oily. After the menopause, decreased estrogen levels also cause skin to lose its plumpness.

The test: Lay your hand flat on a table and pinch the skin on the back, grabbing as much as you can. Hold for one minute, then let it go and watch how long it takes for the skin to return to normal.

1 second or less—8 points
1–2 seconds—6 points
3–4 seconds—4 points
5–10 seconds—3 points
11–30 seconds—2 points
31–45 seconds—1 point

Static balance

Why? Balance relies on ear function, and as you age your hearing gradually deteriorates.

The test: Stand on one leg with the other held in front of you at a 45-degree angle. Place your hands on your hips, close your eyes, and time how long it takes for you to lose your balance. Repeat the test three times, allowing five minutes between each test, and take your best score.

70 seconds or more—8 points
60–69 seconds—6 points
50–59 seconds—4 points
40–49 seconds—3 points
30–39 seconds—2 points
20–29 seconds—1 point

Near vision

Why? Most people notice a significant decline in near vision from their late 40s as the lens of the eye becomes less elastic, resulting in a loss of focusing power.

The test: Position a yard- (meter-) long ruler at your cheekbone directly below your eye so the ruler is horizontal in front of you (if you normally wear glasses or contact lenses for near-sightedness, keep them on, but remove reading glasses). Have the 1-inch mark nearest your face. Hold a business card upright and facing you as far out along the ruler as you can (or have a friend hold it). Slowly move the card towards your eye until the words begin to blur and measure the distance.

3½ in (9 cm) or less—8 points
4–6 in (10–15 cm)—6 points
6½–12 in (16–30 cm)—4 points
12½–24 in (31–60 cm)—3 points
24½–36 in (61–90 cm)—2 points
More than 36 in (90 cm)—1 point

Brain function

Why? A progressive decline in brain function can start in your early 40s, beginning with short-term memory loss and the inability to learn new information.

The test: Try to count back in sevens from 100. If you are under 40, it should take no longer than 20 seconds. If you're between 40 and 60, it should take less than 25 seconds.

20 seconds—8 points
21–25 seconds—4 points
More than 25 seconds—1 point

Lung function

Why? As you age, your lungs are unable to blow out as much air, but regular exercise helps (as does not smoking!).

The test: Place a candle 6 in (15 cm) away from you, get down to the same level as the flame, and then try to blow it out with your mouth open.

Blown out with ease—6 points
All other results—2 points

Your biological age

Add all your answers together to find your score.

56 points or above = a biological age of 20 to 25
51–55 points = a biological age of 26 to 29
46–50 points = a biological age of 30 to 34
41–45 points = a biological age of 35 to 39
36–40 points = a biological age of 40 to 44
28–35 points = a biological age of 45 to 49
21–27 points = a biological age of 50 to 54
16–20 points = a biological age of 55 to 59
11–15 points = a biological age of 60 to 64
0–10 points = a biological age of 65 plus

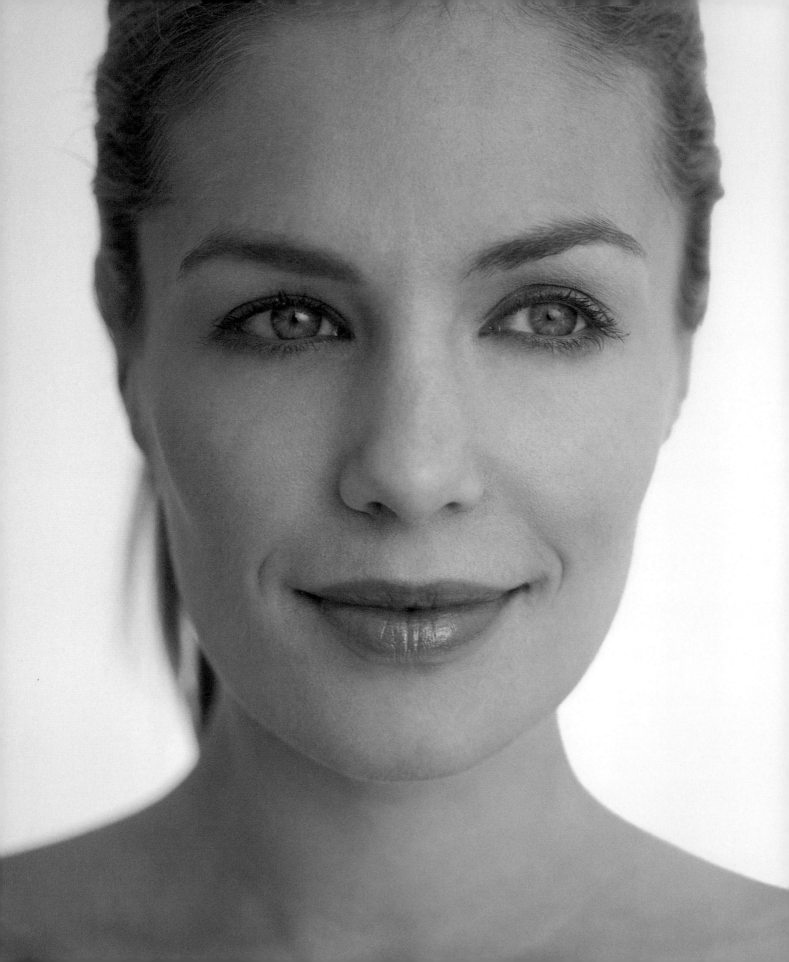

Ageless Face
Keeping your skin glowing

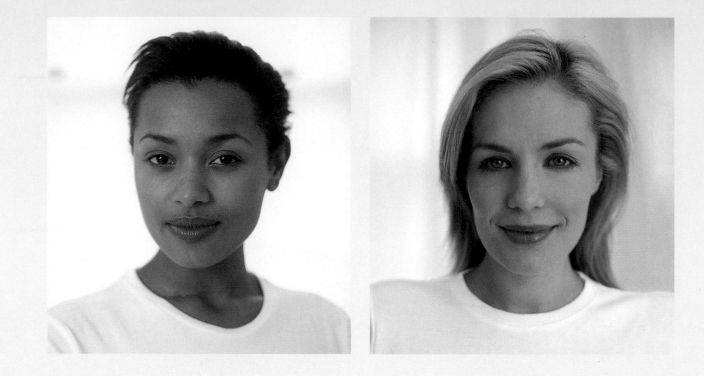

Skin Through the Ages

What follows may make for depressing reading, but modern science means you can now make a significant difference to the way your skin ages—if you just know what to do with it.

20s
This is as good as it gets. You may have pimples in your 20s, but your skin will be in good condition unless you've exposed yourself to some serious sun damage. Cell turnover occurs every 14–25 days. This is when plump new cells work their way up through the layers of your skin, and as they near the surface they flatten out to form lovely fresh skin. Sebum function is also at its peak, meaning your skin may be slightly oily but it feels moist with a healthy glow. Fat under the surface also plumps you up, and fine lines are a distant threat.

What you can do now: When skin is behaving so well on its own it's tempting to skip skincare, but a good regime now will definitely reap future rewards. This is the age of prevention: don't sunbathe to excess, wear a sunscreen every day, eat a healthy diet, drink plenty of water, and it's possible for your skin to stay this way for much longer.

30s
This is when a none-too-shady past can catch up with you. Sun damage is cumulative, so if you've been a sun-worshipper this decade is when pigmentation problems and fine lines will start to show. Your face ages from the top down, so it's your forehead and eyes that see the first signs of wrinkling. Expect a frown line between your eyebrows to appear, too. Your skin may become drier now as sebum production slows, and any dehydration will begin to show up in fine lines. From 30, you start to lose around 1% of collagen and elastin a year, and cell turnover slows to 30 days. You also might notice an increase in skin sensitivity due to stress, working and living in a polluted environment, or drinking alcohol and/or smoking.

What you can do now: You're still on the prevention trail, so swap sunbathing for a fake tan (the only healthy tan there is), eat for good skin (see pages 64–67), and exfoliate daily to enhance the benefits of your moisturizer and make fine lines look less obvious. Wear a sunscreen every day to prevent sun damage from appearing prematurely.

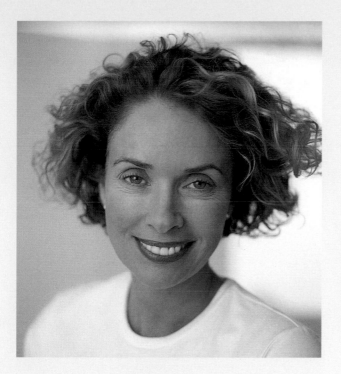

Modern **science** means you can now make a significant **difference** to the way your skin ages—if you just **know** what to do with it.

40s

Many people see a significant change in their skin as they hit 40 (the author certainly did). Cell turnover slows down to 40 days and so does sebum production, good news for anyone with greasy skin but not so great for already dry faces. Dehydration will be far more noticeable in your 40s, emphasizing lines and wrinkles. Expect to see a little sagging around your jaw, and the lines on your forehead, around your eyes, and on your upper lip will either appear or become more noticeable (depending upon how well you've escaped them so far). Your skin will also become thinner, making any age spots (caused by melanin clumping together) much more obvious, and blood capillaries can begin to dilate and leak (rosacea often starts in your 40s—see pages 20–21).

What you can do now: Think increased exfoliation and stimulation to kick-start your skin's renewal, plus use skincare with as many nutrients as possible (see pages 16–17) to regenerate your skin. Fillers made of hyaluronic acid (see page 27) will also make a difference now, as they plump up your skin by adding volume to the amount already there.

50s onwards

This is the decade when wrinkles come out in force, due to a decrease in oil and hormone production levels. This means more prominent under-eye bags (lower eyelid skin thins now, too) and nose to mouth lines. Dehydration increases and cell turnover is now only 45–50 days. If you've been a sunbather, the pigmentation of your skin can now be quite mottled, with many age spots and thread veins. You will also lose the layer of fat under your skin, making your face look thinner.

What you can do now: Encourage slow sebaceous glands and skin renewal by stimulating capillaries with massage (see pages 22–23), which increases blood flow to feed the cells. Use products with vitamins to nourish skin, and silicone-based protectors that seal in moisture. Hydroxy acid in skincare (see page 17) can help refine skin that looks leathery, and fillers will plump out deeper lines.

And the good news: It's not all doom and gloom. Once you're past the menopause, your skin will settle down and you can start to enjoy a clear, glowing complexion again.

The Top Two Skin Sins

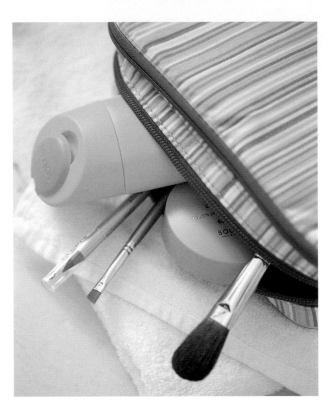

Sun worshipping

Your skin is the most obvious indicator of your age, and by far the best thing you can do to keep looking younger for longer is to protect it from the sun. A massive 80–90% of aging is due to environmental damage, which means much of it doesn't have to happen. Sunbeds are a definite no-go area if you want to avoid premature wrinkles, as their UVA rays are the most aging, penetrating deeper into your skin to break down collagen-forming cells.

No matter how much of a sun worshipper you've been in the past, start protecting your skin now and you won't do any more damage. Dermatologists recommend using a broad-spectrum sunscreen (which protects against both UVA and UVB rays) all year round. Even on wintry days, ultraviolet rays can penetrate your skin, so always choose a moisturizer or foundation with an SPF (sun protection factor) of 15, and during the summer months or on vacation up that to a sunblock with SPF30. Today's sunscreens contain many added anti-aging extras such as antioxidant vitamins and moisturizers, but the most important ingredient is the SPF—so if buying basic means you can afford to use it every day, the basic option is more beneficial to your skin than any posh-sounding additives.

Some sensitive skins can't take the chemicals used in sunscreens, so if you're someone whose skin irritates easily, go for a mineral sunscreen (which contains zinc oxide or titanium dioxide). They create a barrier to reflect light away without being absorbed into your skin. And don't forget to apply sunscreen to your neck, as the skin there is thinner than your face so it ages more quickly.

Smoking

At least the sun provides you with bone-strengthening vitamin D, but there's nothing to be said in favor of skin's other archenemy. We now know that for every 10 years of smoking, the face of a 20-a-day smoker ages 14 years, which means a smoker in their 40s could have as many wrinkles as a non-smoker in their 60s!

Here's why:

* Smoking reduces the production of collagen by up to 40%. Aging already reduces the amount of collagen we produce, and smoking just speeds up this process.
* The accumulated nicotine in your body deprives skin cells of vital oxygen, and smoking also reduces blood flow to the skin, robbing it of even more nutrients.
* When an organ is under attack (i.e., your lungs), your body diverts essential vitamins away from your skin to help.
* Smoking adversely affects the nerve endings in the skin, causing sensitivity.
* Smoke has a drying effect on the skin, causing dehydration and eventually wrinkles. Add to this the squinting and puckering that goes on during smoking and you're creating even more lines, which will eventually become permanent.
* Smoking reduces the body's store of vitamin A (which protects against skin damage) and vitamin C (which protects against aging free radicals). Giving up may be hard to do, but the benefits are almost instant. Within eight hours, nicotine and carbon monoxide levels in your body are cut in half, and in just two weeks you'll see an obvious improvement in your skin's color (no more dull, gray days) and texture. You know it makes sense.

Your skin is the most obvious indicator of your age, and by far the **best thing** you can do to keep looking younger for longer is to **protect it** from the sun.

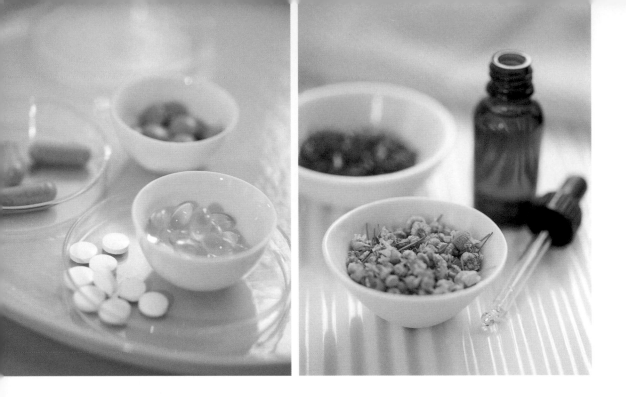

Ingredients to the Rescue

Did you know that some anti-aging skincare products contain very few ingredients that have much impact on your skin? However, if you buy something packed with the goodies listed below, your skin will instantly feel the benefits. Become an ingredient reader, and also look out for skincare brands labeled "cosmeceuticals" (meaning cosmetics with pharmacological activity), as these will have a more significant effect on your skin than any cosmetic cream (see Directory).

Antioxidants

These are what you need to fight (and even reverse) free-radical damage. Free radicals are unstable oxygen molecules with only one electron, so they must scavenge other molecules for their missing one. This causes the other molecules to become unstable, setting up a process that damages cell function resulting in a loss of elasticity, slackness, discoloration, and wrinkles.

What to look for: Green tea, grape seed (a superior ingredient that also enhances any SPF in the product), fumitory, licorice, ascorbic acid, tocopherol, retinyl palmitate, ginkgo biloba, and Japanese alder.

Anti-enzyme agents

These protect vital structures in the skin and also help maintain skin firmness and elasticity.

What to look for: Echinacea, hydrocotyl, grape seed extract, flavenoids, and green tea.

Anti-inflammatories

These soothe, calm, and reduce redness (so are great for acne and rosacea sufferers), and also stop itching.

What to look for: Licorice, Canadian willow herb, green tea, silanediol salicylate, methylsilanol mannuronate, sage and red clover, avena sativa, cucumber, and camomile.

Cellular stimulants

These encourage healthy skin cells and also stimulate cell growth and activity.

What to look for: Ergothioneine, vitamin A, echinacea, sage and red clover, wheat germ extract, bioflavenoids, and corallina officinalis.

Become an **ingredient** reader, and look out for skincare brands labeled **"cosmeceuticals"** (cosmetics with pharmacological activity).

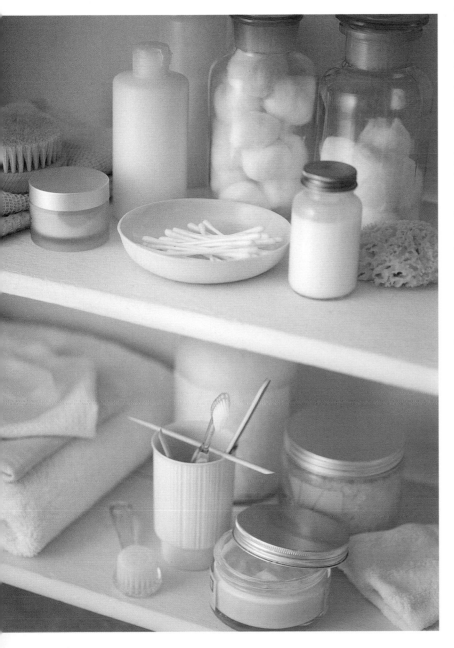

Exfoliants

A must for older skins, to stimulate cell renewal and remove dead skin cells from the surface. Regular use also improves penetration of any other active ingredients and helps reduce fine lines, pigmentation, and dryness.

What to look for: Hydroxy acids (a word of caution: these are great for sun damage, but a too-strong pH can cause sensitivity, so for best results consult a skincare specialist—see Directory), vitamins, enzymes, and abrasives.

Emollients and protectors

These remain on the skin's surface to act as a barrier and keep skin soft and smooth. Beware the cheapest emollients, mineral oil and lanolin, which can clog the skin and cause irritation.

What to look for: Cyclomethicone, phospholipids, shea butter, algae extract, cyclopentasiloxane, and retinyl palmitate.

Vitamins

Taking vitamin supplements may benefit the rest of you, but they won't do much for your skin, as your body considers it your least important organ. Much better are vitamins in a product, which go straight to where they're needed.

What to look for: Vitamin A reverses sun damage and stimulates collagen (retinyl palmitate and retinol). Vitamin B6 aids healing (panthenol). Vitamin E works as an antioxidant and protector (tocopherol and tocopheryl acetate). Vitamin P is great for rosacea, as it's an anti-inflammatory and also improves capillary strength (grape seed extract, ginkgo, and raspberry). Vitamin C is a powerful antioxidant which also stimulates collagen and brightens the skin (ascorbic acid and ascorbyl palmitate).

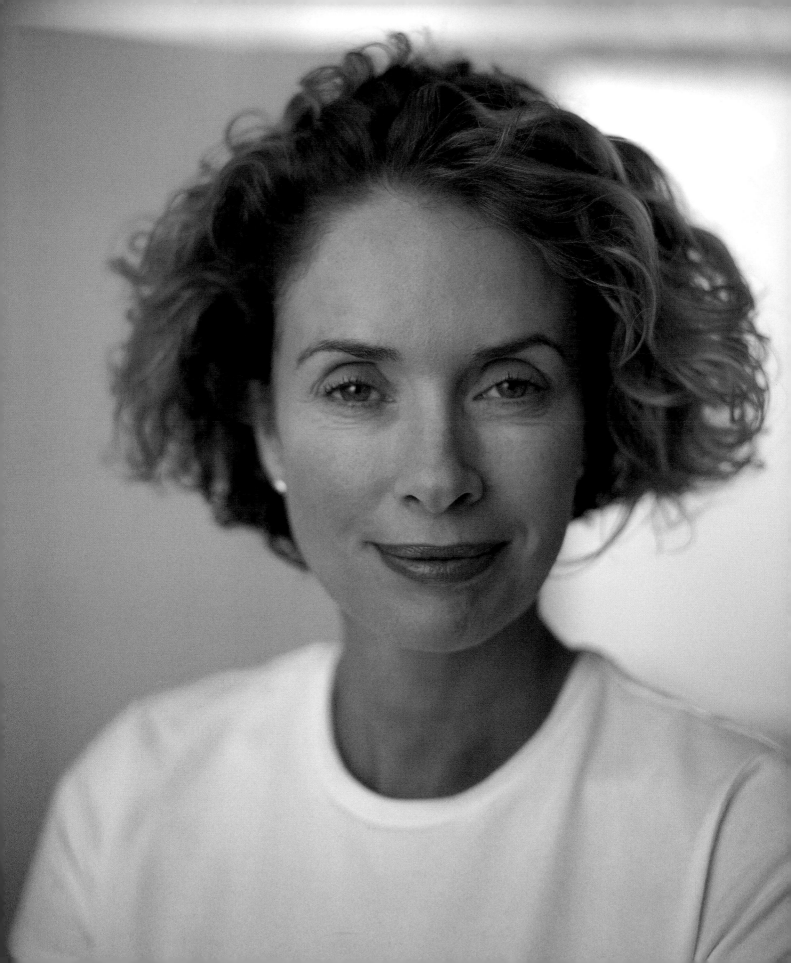

Eva Fraser's Facial Fitness

Seeing your face begin to droop is no fun, but Eva Fraser is convinced that with just a little effort this gradual deterioration needn't happen. She believes that the muscles in the face can be retrained like any other muscles to become firm and strong again. With just 10–15 minutes of facial exercising a day, Eva promises you will improve the structure of your face and take years off your looks. Nose to mouth lines will lessen, upper cheeks will be lifted and fuller, your jawline will be firmer, and your eyelids will be stronger and lifted. Below are four easy-to-follow exercises from Eva's facial workout (find the rest in her best-selling book—see Directory).

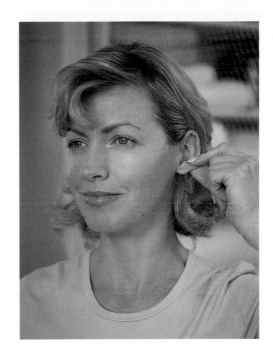

Eyelid lift

1 Raise your eyebrows as high as you can in one slow movement.
2 At the same time, open your eyes as wide as possible.
3 Hold for a count of 10 without blinking, then relax.
4 Now close your eyes.
5 Again raise your eyebrows as above.
6 You should feel a stretch up with your eyebrows, and at the same time a stretch down with your lids.
7 Hold for a count of 10.
8 Lower your eyebrows and open your lids.
9 Repeat once.

Mouth corner lift

1 Begin with your mouth closed. Your lips should sit together without tension.
2 Move one side at a time and keep the other side of your mouth still.
3 Smile up to the outer corner of your eye in four movements. Half-close your eye.
4 Hold for a count of six, feeling a lift from jawline to the corner of your eye.
5 Return slowly in four movements.
6 Repeat twice on each side, making sure all movements are made from your mouth corner.

Lower face lift

1 Stretch your chin up so you are holding the front of your neck taut.
2 Draw your lower lip up over your top lip.
3 Smile toward the middle of your ear in six steps.
4 Now jut your chin slightly more forward and up, feeling a stretch along your jawline towards your earlobes.
5 Hold for a count of six and release slowly.
6 Repeat once.

Ear massage

This stimulates the flow of blood to your face.
1 With your index fingers and thumbs, hold the top rim of your ears and lift slightly upwards. With small rotations between fingers and thumbs, massage this area.
2 Move down around the rim of the ears, pulling the ears out gently and massaging. Continue like this all around the rim of the ears.
3 When you reach the lobes, pull them down slightly and massage again.
4 Now work back upwards to the top of the rim and repeat the above for about a minute.
5 Lastly, using small, quick circular movements, massage all the crevices of the ears. The pads of the index fingers (not the tips) are best for this.

Why is my Face Red?

One in 20 people has rosacea, which causes facial flushing and redness, yet most of us don't know what it is. Many people with rosacea assume they have either sensitive skin or acne. This is especially worrying because if rosacea is left untreated it becomes progressively worse. There's no cure, but you can keep it under control if you know what to do.

What does it look like?

Symptoms of rosacea include mild to constant flushing and acne-type breakouts. You may get a sudden sensitivity to

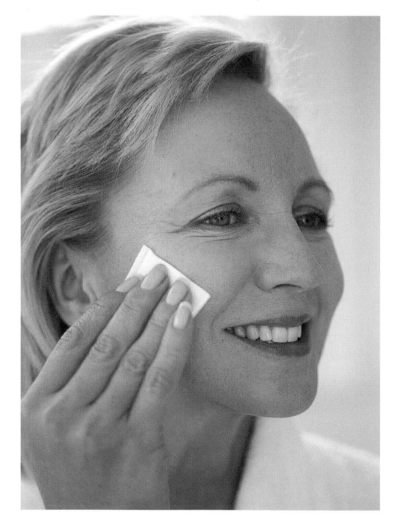

products you've used for ages, and during a flare-up (which will last around 30 minutes) your skin may burn and itch. The skin on your nose, chin, and forehead are most affected and can become sore and swollen.

What causes it?

Rosacea is an abnormality of facial blood vessels and its most likely cause is genetic, with 40% of sufferers saying someone else in their family has it too. Symptoms usually start around age 30 to 50 and, although hormones don't cause rosacea, if you're already genetically prone, hormonal changes (such as during the menopause) can aggravate the condition.

What happens during an attack?

Too much blood is pumped through your capillaries, causing them to stretch and lose their elasticity. This makes them unable to work properly, so the capillaries become overloaded and your skin goes red. Your lymphatic system can't take away all this extra fluid and it builds up in the surrounding tissue, causing inflammation and swelling.

What brings on an attack?

Rosacea-prone skin is stimulated very easily by the following common triggers.

* Hot liquids such as coffee or tea; alcohol (especially red wine); spicy foods; and histamine-producing foods such as tomatoes. Keep a food diary so you can work out exactly what triggers an attack for you.
* Stress, as it stimulates your system, causing increased capillary action.
* Changes or extremes in temperature (winter can be the worst time for rosacea sufferers, as they alternate between the cold outdoors and heated indoors).
* Intense exercise that stimulates the skin, such as running or hot yoga. Much better options are regular hatha yoga, walking, and Pilates.
* Smoking, which depletes the body's vitamin C levels, causing weaker capillaries.

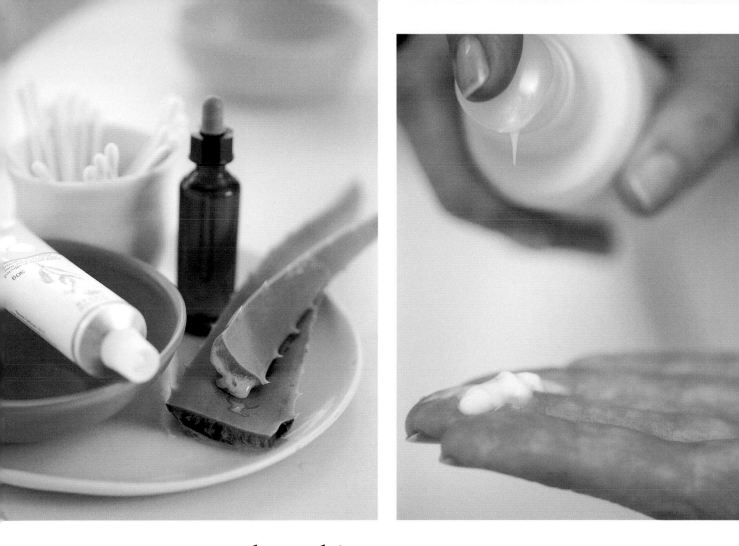

The **best thing** you can do for your skin is create a barrier between it and the **outside world**.

What can I do to improve it?

Avoid your triggers as much as possible, and practice slowing down (see pages 116–117), because reducing your stress levels can have a massive effect on your skin. It's also well worth seeing an experienced skin therapist (see Directory), who can recommend the right products. You can seriously improve your skin just by knowing what to avoid. Your enemies include any face scrubs and peels; alcohol; fragrance (the number one sensitizer in products); witch hazel, menthol, peppermint and eucalyptus oils (which are all astringent); and oil-based creams that feel greasy on your skin. The best thing you can do for your skin is create a barrier between it and the outside world. You should also keep well moisturized to prevent water loss, and protect your skin from the sun all year round with a mineral-based sunscreen to deflect capillary-damaging sunlight.

Other rosacea-friendly ingredients to look out for include aloe vera, allantoin (from the comfrey plant), and arnica, which are all great anti-inflammatories; red clover and red raspberry, which strengthen capillaries; licorice, which is both an anti-inflammatory and an antioxidant; and camomile and lavender, which are soothing. The best way to treat pimples is with a dab of tea tree oil applied on a Q-tip. As for makeup, a great choice for rosacea sufferers is mineral makeup, as it's non-pore-blocking and oil-free, minimum allergy risk, and anti-inflammatory (see Directory).

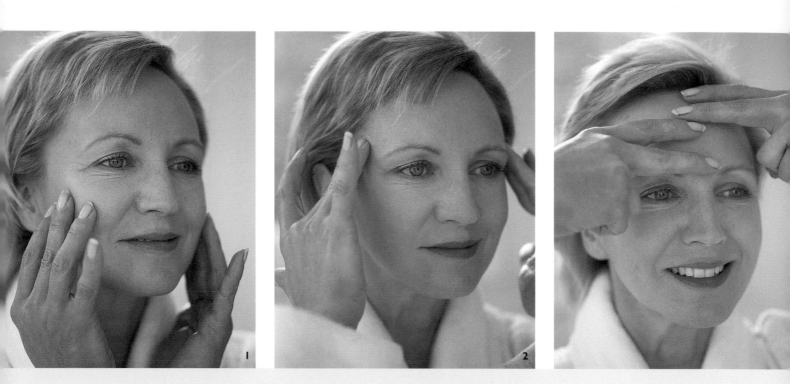

1

2

Anti-aging Facial

Massaging your face can significantly improve your skin's health. Stimulating blood circulation brings an increased supply of oxygen and nutrients to the skin, boosting cell regeneration while removing waste substances that can cause skin to become sluggish and dull. Improved oil production also aids skin protection and promotes a healthy glow. Lastly, massage will relieve tension and fatigue, and relaxed facial features mean less obvious lines and wrinkles. Bring tired skin back to life with these easy massage movements developed by Candice Gardner and Kelly Quinn at the International Dermal Institute (see Directory).

First apply moisturizer or serum to your skin to ensure it's a little slippery—the last thing you want is to drag or over-stretch your skin. Repeat each movement 3–6 times, depending upon how much time you have.

1 Facial tapping
What it does: Stimulates blood circulation and skin oxygenation.
The massage: Using the index, middle, and ring fingers of both hands flat on your face, drum all over with a light tapping movement.

2 Tissue release
What it does: Releases facial tension.
The massage: Starting on your forehead, use the fingertips of both hands to push the skin tissue up in a small semi-circular rotation toward the hairline. Allow to drop naturally. Work over your entire face, pushing upward on each movement.

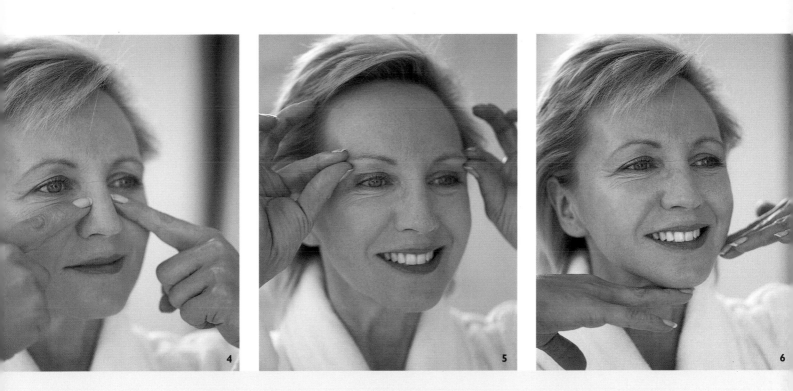

3 Forehead zigzag

What it does: Smooths lines and wrinkles.

The massage: Place the middle and index fingers of both hands on your forehead and slide them toward the center in a zigzag motion so your fingers pass each other.

4 Sinus drain

What it does: Reduces skin puffiness and promotes tissue detoxification.

The massage: Halfway up your nose where the cheekbone meets the nasal bone is a small hollow which, when pressed, may feel tender. Apply pressure using your middle finger for a count of five and release, then slide your fingers across the cheekbone toward your ears to drain.

At the corners of your nose, press back into the cheekbone to find a second hollow that may also be tender. Apply pressure for a count of five and release, then slide your fingers under the cheekbone to your ears to drain.

5 Eyebrow pinch

What it does: Releases eye strain and forehead tension.

The massage: Gently pinch along your brow bone using thumb and forefinger, starting in the center of your eyebrows.

6 Jawline roll patting

What it does: Stimulates and lifts the jaw tissue.

The massage: Using the backs of your hands, sweep alternate hands up your neck toward your jaw, moving from one ear to the other.

Five-second fix

Use a toner after your morning cleanse to rev up blood and lymphatic circulation, which becomes stagnant during sleep—the cause of that first-thing-in-the-morning dull complexion.

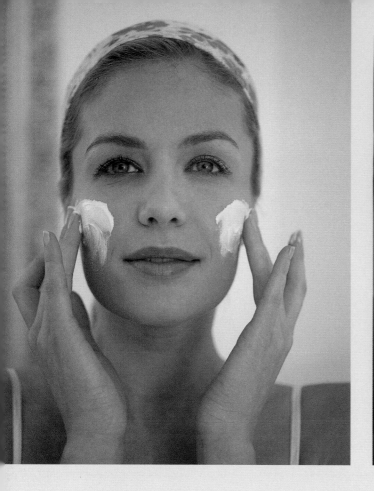

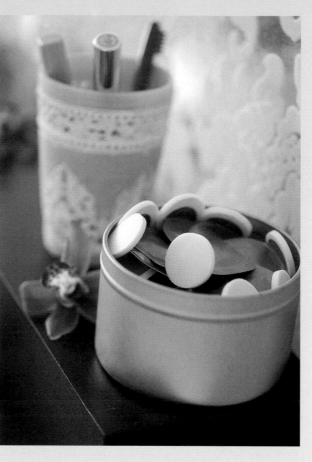

Ten Tips for Aging Well

The International Dermal Institute (see Directory) has the following expert advice for keeping your skin looking younger for longer.

1 Always use a broad-spectrum (meaning it protects from both UVA and UVB rays) sunblock with a minimum SPF15 all year round. Between 80 and 90% of all skin aging is blamed on UV exposure, so it's essential to protect yourself outside even when the sun's not shining.

2 Exfoliate 2–3 times a week to encourage new skin cells to form and help these fresh cells travel to the skin's surface more quickly. Exfoliation also helps fine lines look less visible by smoothing the surface and giving your skin a glow.

3 Rather than apply one layer of thick gooey cream, your skin will be kept more supple and better protected if you layer your moisturizing products. That means a hydrating spritz sealed in with a protective moisturizer and finished off with that all-important broad-spectrum sunblock.

4 Avoid using harsh products (anything with a strong smell, or even a whiff of antiseptic!) or harsh treatments on your skin. They both encourage sensitivity and dehydration, leading to premature aging. Constantly changing your skincare, or mixing and matching from many ranges, can also sensitize your skin, so find a brand that suits you and stick with it.

5 Drink lots of water all year round (and not just in summer), as this not only keeps your skin well hydrated but also flushes out waste toxins.

Exfoliating 2–3 times a week helps fine lines look less visible by smoothing the surface and giving your skin a glow.

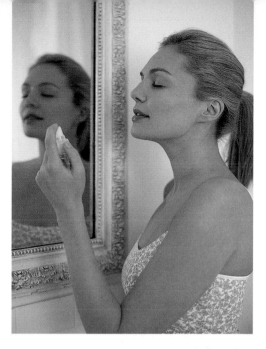

6 Stop smoking immediately. Not only do waste toxins give you a yellow or gray complexion, but nicotine also deprives the skin of vital oxygen (see page 14 for what else smoking does to your skin).

7 As we get older, essential vitamins in our diet are diverted to the body's other organs, so choose skincare products to supplement your skin. Anti-aging vitamins to look out for are vitamins A, B5, E, P (bioflavenoids), and C (see pages 16–17 for more on wonder ingredients for aging skin).

8 Get plenty of sleep, as your skin repairs itself overnight when your body's energy is no longer needed for day-to-day living (see pages 96–97 for what else sleep can do for you).

9 Cut down your alcohol consumption. Alcohol raises blood pressure, causing your capillaries to dilate. In time they will weaken, leading to permanent redness and sensitivity. The chemicals alcohol produces also cause dehydration and destroy minerals needed for daily skin functions (caffeine in tea and coffee cause dehydration, too).

10 Learn to deal with the stress in your life with relaxation techniques (see pages 116–117 for ideas on how to slow down), as stress and unhappiness are major causes of age acceleration.

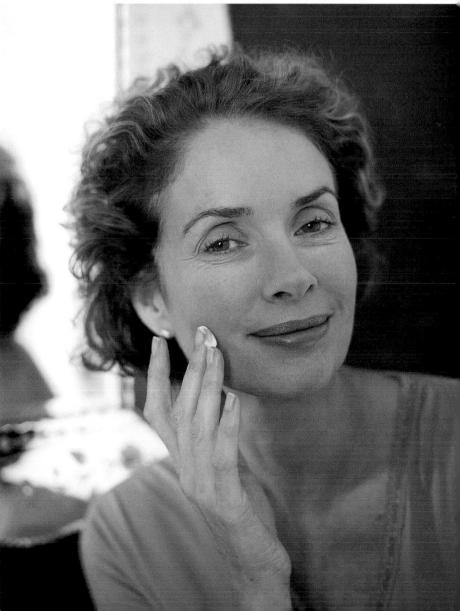

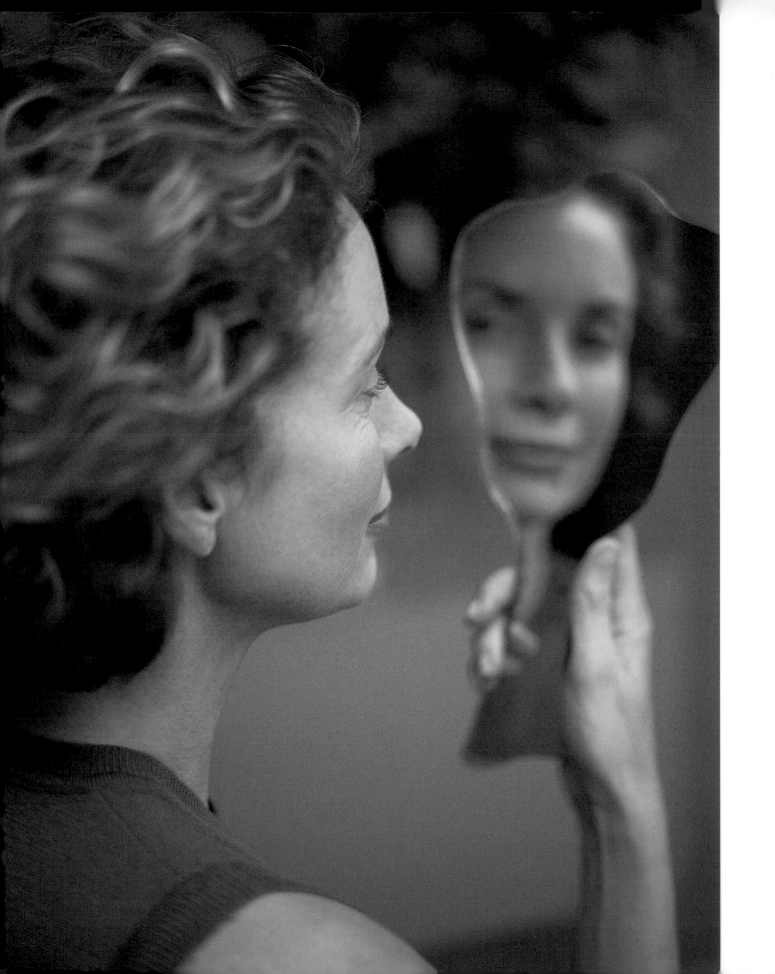

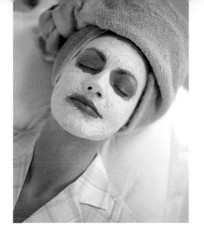

When Nature Needs a Little Help

With the introduction of less scary, knife-free procedures, cosmetic surgery is becoming more and more popular for reversing signs of aging. Even with the following non-invasive treatments, it's still vital you choose a qualified cosmetic surgeon (check yours is registered with a professional body—see Directory). And make sure you know exactly what you're getting into beforehand, including possible side effects and recovery time. Lastly, trust your instincts. If you feel uneasy, then go elsewhere.

Botox

Purified botulinum toxin is injected into specific facial muscles in very tiny amounts to freeze them. Most commonly used for frown lines, forehead lines, and crow's feet, the toxin attaches itself to the muscle so it can't move when you frown or squint. Expect a little bruising and tiny red pinpricks where the needle went in, which will fade in a few days. "Freezing" happens gradually over the next few days and wears off after three to six months. You need to stay upright for three to four hours after treatment, moving the injected muscles regularly to disperse the toxin, and don't fly for 24 hours.

Fillers

More injections, depositing a substance under the skin to smooth irregularities such as wrinkles, pits, and scars. Fillers firm facial contours and re-plump lips and cheeks.

Collagen was the first filler on the market, but has lost favor because the protein substance (most often derived from cattle) can cause an allergic reaction. For this reason, patients must be tested prior to treatment. A local anesthetic can be used to minimize discomfort from the injection needle, and effects last three to nine months.

Hyaluronic acid is the most popular filler as it's free from animal products, so less likely to cause a reaction. The most common are Restylane and Perlane, used for plumping lines, folds, and thinning lips. Results last longer than collagen—six to nine months, and up to 12—so expect to pay more.

Body sculpturing involves removing fat from a plumper part of your body (think hips, buttocks, or thighs) and injecting it somewhere that needs plumping up (such as sunken cheeks, deep folds, and thinning lips). This is a more complicated treatment performed in an outpatient clinic, so recovery time can take up to a week, with results lasting between three and six months.

Chemical peels

Effective at treating sun damage, age spots, and wrinkles, peels also stimulate the production of collagen in the skin. A chemical such as alpha-hydroxy or glycolic acid is applied (for between 2 and 10 minutes), which causes surface skin to shed and be replaced with a clearer, less mottled layer. The immediate result is similar to sunburn, and then peels off over a period of up to five days. A mild peel is all that's needed to treat fine lines and wrinkles, but a medium-depth peel is most effective for more serious skin damage (this has an increased recovery time of 7–14 days).

Microdermabrasion

Less dramatic than a peel, this technique uses very small crystals (such as aluminum salts) to remove the outermost layer of skin—and the superficial imperfections on it. The procedure takes about 30 minutes and your skin will look pinker (but brighter) afterwards. Great for irregular pigmentation and fine lines, microdermabrasion is not intensive enough to tackle deeper skin damage. A course of treatments is recommended.

PS After any treatment that exfoliates the skin deeply, it's highly recommended that you use a sunscreen every day—but then you do that already, don't you?

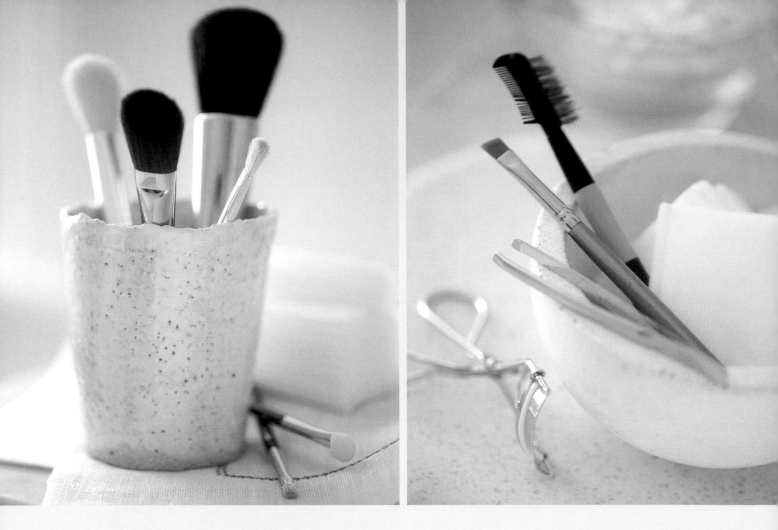

Age-defying Makeup Tricks

* As you age, less is definitely more, but don't make the mistake of going totally bare-faced. Women who wear makeup often have less environmentally damaged skin.
* If you're still wearing the same makeup you did 10 years ago, it's worth booking an appointment with a makeup artist at your favorite beauty counter. They'll be able to demonstrate the latest products and show you how to make the very best of your face.
* Start using a foundation that contains an SPF, vitamins, and antioxidants, to protect your skin from future signs of age.
* Apply base with your fingers or a foundation brush rather than a sponge, which will deposit too much, making fine lines and open pores more visible.

* Avoid heavy, matte foundations or powder-based products, which can settle into fine lines. Instead, go for a "light-diffusing" or "line-smoothing" liquid base to give a luminous finish while still hiding what you don't want to show.
* Mineral makeup is great for sensitive skin conditions, and also contains skin benefits such as a natural non-irritating SPF and time-release antioxidants. It's also non-pore-blocking so won't add to hormonal acne problems, while giving very good coverage for age-related imperfections. (See Directory.)
* Instead of shimmery face powders, go for a little pearly highlighter on brow and cheekbones to give your face a lift, and add radiance that may no longer come naturally!

Choose **softer** versions of the more intense colors you normally wear, or go for **neutral shades** like nude, peach, rose, and brown.

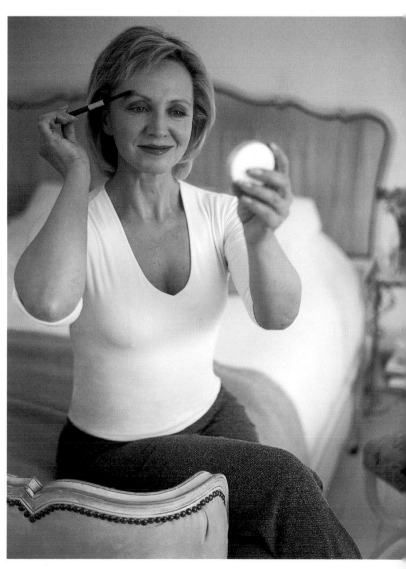

* To give your face the illusion of lift, choose a foundation one shade lighter than your normal one. Apply it around the entire eye socket and on top of your cheekbones to create lightness across the center of your face.

* A flattering blush can take attention away from your eyes (and the crow's feet around them), and bring back a youthful glow. For a fresh look use a mauve- or rose-based color, which will mimic the natural flush of your cheeks. And remember, blusher isn't for contouring, so use a light hand to apply just over the apples of your cheeks.

* Strong colors look hard on older skins and draw attention to places you may not desire to highlight after a certain age! Instead, choose softer versions of the more intense colors you normally wear, or switch to neutral shades like nude, peach, rose, and brown.

* Shimmery eyeshadows will only highlight laughter lines and crepey eyelids, so avoid them at all costs.

* Nothing opens up eyes more than curling your eyelashes. Also, match mascara to your lashes (black mascara on brown lashes is very aging).

* Wax eye pencils will drag your eye all over the place, so choose a cream-to-powder liner, which is easier to apply and more long-lasting.

* Keep your brows well defined to stop them from looking sparse. Use a soft pencil (blunt the end on the back of your hand first) or matte eyeshadow applied with a stiff brush, and choose a color one shade lighter than your brows.

For tips on making up your lips, see pages 42–43.

Anti-aging Secrets of the Rich and Famous

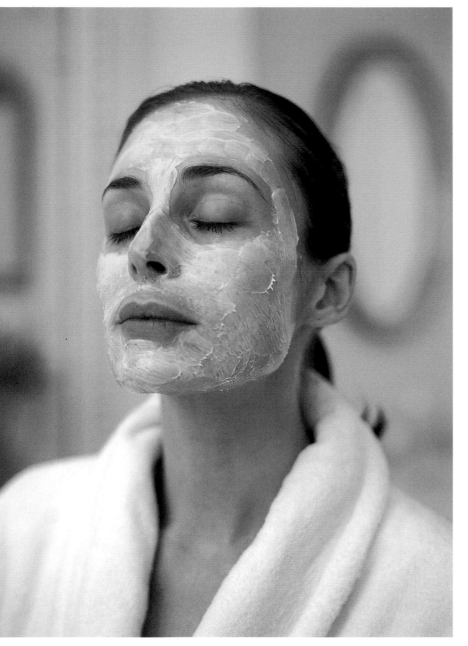

Intense pulsed light (IPL)

Also known as photorejuvenation, this non-invasive procedure treats pigmentation marks; redness, including broken veins; and irregular skin texture. Unlike more aggressive laser resurfacing, you can go back to the office with only a slight redness to give away where you've spent your lunch hour. It can't be done over a tan or self-tanning products as there's a risk of burning, and you need to avoid sunbathing and wear a sunblock during your course of treatments. A cooling gel is applied before the treatment head is moved slowly over your face. While not exactly painful, each light pulse feels as if your skin has been gently snapped with a rubber band. And the bigger the target, the sharper the snap! Afterwards, skin is glowing and brown spots are darker, but "fall off" as you cleanse your face a few days later. A session costs from $200 (depending upon where you go) and, although you can expect to see improvements after one, the recommended course is between four and six. (See Directory.)

Skin supplements

These are food supplement tablets that are taken daily to work from the inside out to improve your skin's thickness, elasticity, and moisture levels. The tablets contain skin-friendly ingredients such as marine extracts, active proteins, silica, and vitamin C, which all promote the natural rejuvenation of your skin. Results can be seen after three months, not just on your face but all over your body, and you can expect

Eyelash extensions are just about the **most flattering** beauty treatment you can have.

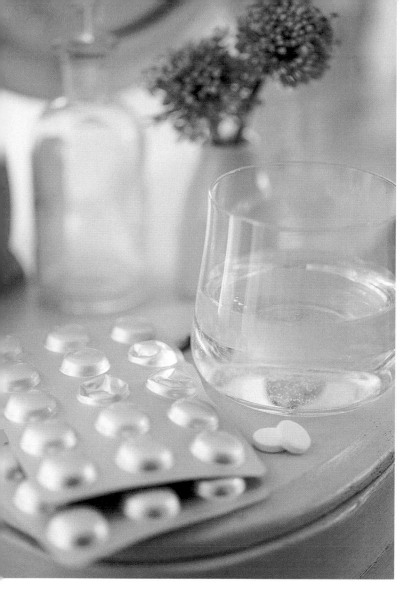

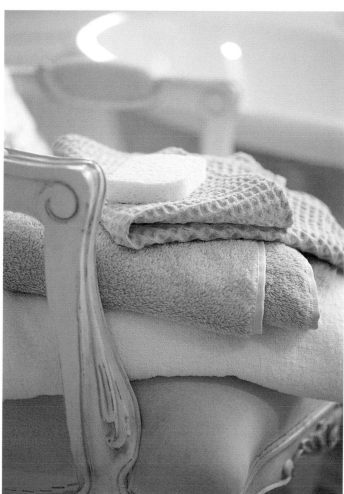

signs of aging such as fine lines, age spots, and dilated capillaries to be visibly reduced. Your skin will look brighter and smoother too, and the author also got a couple of compliments about how young she looked for her age! These results don't come cheap, with a month's supply costing from $15 (depending upon the brand you choose), but there's clinical evidence that these work and, of course, they're far cheaper than surgery. (See Directory.)

Eyelash extensions

Unlike traditional false lashes, these are single lashes that are painstakingly attached to your real ones rather than your skin (just as hair extensions are attached to the hair, not the scalp). This means they look completely natural and last 6–12 weeks, shedding as your natural eyelashes do. Each treatment attaches from 40 lashes per eye, taking roughly one minute per lash. It's just about the most flattering beauty treatment you can have, and as the lashes are curled, you can say goodbye to mascara, not to mention any other eye makeup.

Prices aren't cheap, starting from around $250 for a full set, but ask about a complimentary top-up a week later in case any of the "anchor" lashes have fallen off. Give your new lashes the longest life possible by not letting any water, skincare, or makeup near them for 24 hours, and from then on, cleansing around your eyes very carefully. And sleep on your back, if at all possible! (See Directory.)

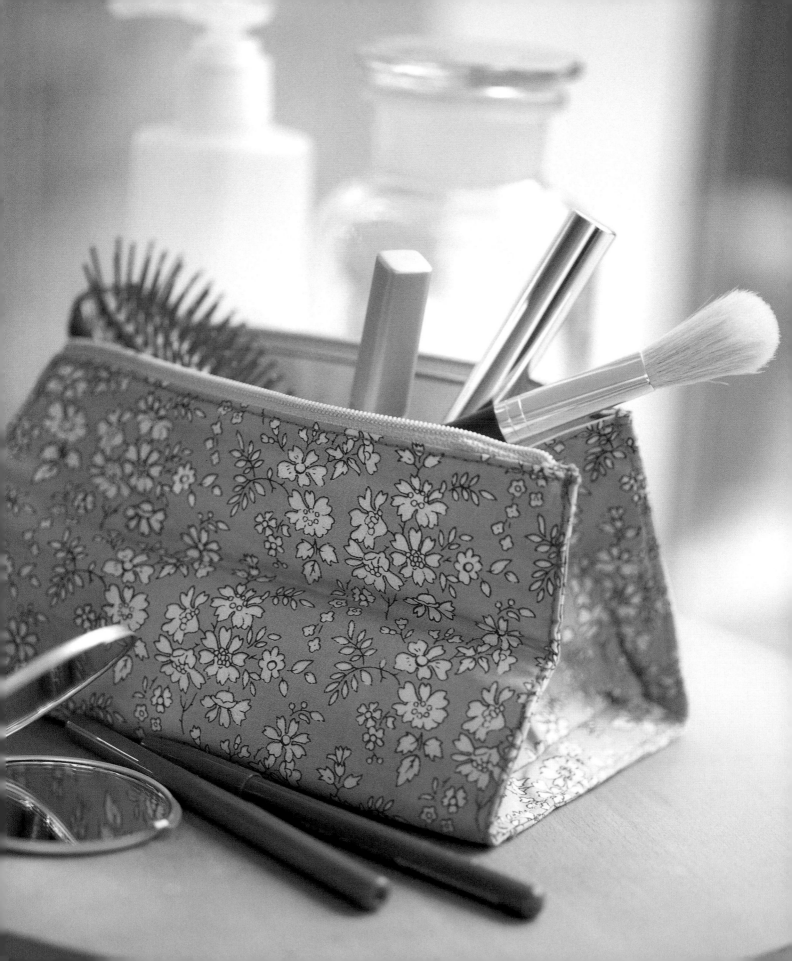

Making up Through the Ages

Daniel Sandler, makeup artist to Kristin Scott Thomas and Joanna Lumley, says, "Makeup should always be sheer, regardless of your age. Always be subtle with application and look for formulations that suit your skin. If you've not changed your base in 20 years, have a look at today's new formulations, which make a massive difference to your skin."

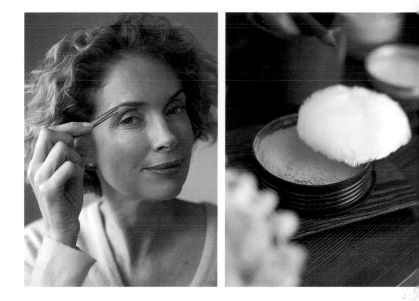

20s
Foundation: There's no need to wear base unless you have an uneven skintone, and look for an oil-free liquid or stick formula with added SPF, as you probably have slightly greasy skin. Use loose powder to set it in place.
Blusher: Powders and stains are longer-lasting than most creams, which can move around during the day.
Eyes: You can wear anything from glitters to shimmers to bold color, so make the most of it while you can!
Lips and nails: Wearing high-fashion colors means it makes sense to buy inexpensive brands. You'll be into a new trend in a few months, so splashing out is a waste of money.

30s and 40s
Foundation: Skin is starting to look a little drier from sun and stress, so look for a liquid base that contains moisturizers and an SPF, but is still light in texture and invisible on the skin. Avoid using loose powder unless it's non-dehydrating, and steer clear of shimmery powders as they can settle into lines. You'll probably need a liquid concealer under your eyes (a light-reflecting one in a slightly yellowy tone is most flattering), and avoid any powder in this area as it enhances fine lines.
Blusher: You can still use powders, but beware going too brown in shade. Much more flattering is a pink or peach over the apples of your cheeks to give a healthy glow. You can also highlight cheekbones with just a touch of shimmer.
Eyes: Apply a little foundation on lids to hide veins and help eyeshadows last and blend well. Avoid using glitter all over the lids—a dot at the center is enough.
Lips: Color is a personal choice, but avoid shimmery shades as they are often dry in texture.

50s onwards
Foundation: Avoid oil-free formulations, as you need extra help with moisturizing now. Liquid or creamy formulations will flatter; they should also be light-reflecting, but not too shimmery. Steer clear of stick foundations, which tend to dry out your skin, and too much powder, which can look floury.
Blusher: Use long-lasting creams that won't budge, as powders will be too dry, making your skin look dull.
Eyes: Avoid dark, matte shades all over the lids and go for sheer delicates. If you want extra definition, use a soft liner pencil close to your lash line and smudge with a finger. You may have a few gray hairs in your brows, but don't over-darken, as this just looks scary. Update your look with a flattering color like lilac, which brightens the whites and makes the iris color stand out. And definitely avoid glitter—you aren't your daughter!
Lips: Avoid too much gloss as it will run into creases, and don't use very dark shades as they will make your face look hard. If your lips aren't as plump as they used to be, line with a soft, neutral shade pencil, fill in with color, and use a dot of gloss just in the center of your lower lip.

Eyes: Smoothing, Lightening, and De-puffing

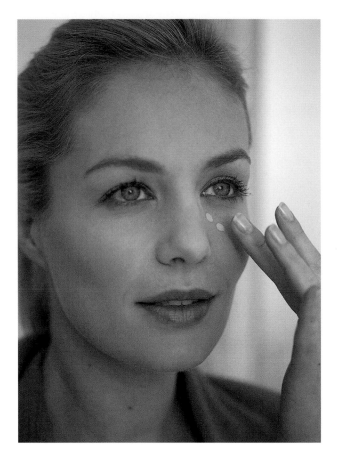

Smoothing lines

The skin around your eyes is 10 times thinner than the rest of your face. Add to that the fact that your eyes are the most expressive part of your face, and it's no surprise wrinkles show up here first. The skin is also low on natural lubrication, which makes it very receptive to cosmetic creams, and for once the idea of buying a separate eye product isn't just a clever marketing ploy. The thinner skin around your eyes really can't absorb thick-textured creams, so your normal night or day cream will be too heavy (and could cause puffiness). Instead, invest in a separate eye product packed with anti-aging vitamins, and only use a blob the size of a small pea for both eyes to avoid overload. For best results, use an eye cream or serum at night to prevent dehydration,

and an eye cream or gel (preferably with an SPF) in the morning to stimulate circulation and reduce puffiness. Use your ring finger to pat gently onto the skin over crow's feet and around the eye contour, avoiding eyelids.

Dark circles

Dark circles can happen at any age, but become more noticeable as skin thins and blood entering the vessels under your eyes shows through. The most common reason for dark circles is lack of sleep, although stress, a food intolerance (which can be triggered by stress), and smoking can also cause problems. And don't ignore genetics. If your mother has dark circles, you may well have inherited them, too. The first line of defense is to drink plenty of water to flush out toxins, and cut down on alcohol and salty food. You can also try avoiding wheat and cow's milk, which are the most common food-intolerance triggers. Luckily, light-diffusing concealers work wonders at disguising dark circles. And application is foolproof if you bear in mind that less is more.

Drop your chin and look up at yourself in a mirror so you can see the darkest area. This is where you need to apply a line of concealer, preferably with a fine brush. Then work quickly to blend over the entire dark area, being careful not to overlap onto lighter skin—or your camouflage work will have a highlighting effect instead.

Puffy eyes

Puffiness is caused by trapped fluid in the tissues under your eyes, and is usually worse in the morning as fluid collects overnight. Eyebags after a boozy night out or a good cry are common, but if you suffer regularly you may have a food intolerance. Again, common triggers are wheat and cow's milk products (including cheese and cottage cheese), plus citrus fruits, eggs, and nuts. You should also cut down on salt, which increases water retention in all parts of the body. And beware hidden salt. You may be aware that pre-packaged foods are high in salt, but did you know that mass-produced breakfast cereals often contain more salt than a bag of potato chips? Puffy eyes can also be a sign of sensitivity, so it's worth switching cosmetic brands you use daily to see if that makes a difference. And make sure you're not overloading your eyes with a too-rich cream.

No-cost remedies for reducing puffiness

* Wrap an ice cube in plastic wrap and hold it over the area for a few minutes, as this will stimulate blood vessels and help the flow of toxins. Stainless-steel teaspoons kept in the fridge all night will also do the trick.
* Place slices of raw potato on closed eyes for five minutes.
* The tannic acid in black tea is great for reducing swelling. Soak two teabags in cold water and place over your eyes for 10 minutes.
* Tap the under-eye area lightly and quickly with your middle finger, moving from the inner corner outwards and back again.

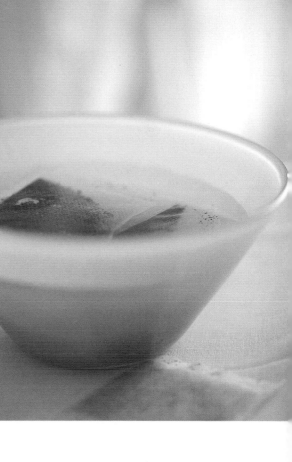

Just as exercising
your body makes
it more flexible,
exercising the
muscles that
control the lenses
of **your eyes**
will also help
strengthen them.

Anti-aging for Eyes

The lenses of your eyes lose elasticity as you age, which impairs your ability to adjust your focus quickly to objects nearby. As they get older, most people can still see distances, but if reading the small print starts to become a problem, it's time for an eye test. You should have an eye test every two years, whether or not you currently wear glasses or contacts.

Exercises for eyes

Just as exercising your body makes it more flexible, exercising the muscles that control the lenses of your eyes will also help strengthen them.

* Hold out your thumb at arm's length and move it first in circles and then in large figures of eight. As you do so, follow your thumb with your eyes, bringing it closer to you and then moving it further away.
* Avoid computer-stuck eyes by switching your focus regularly. Look past your computer every 10 minutes or so and focus on something at least 6 ft (2 m) away. If you're not by a window, give yourself a plant or picture to look at.

Sun protection

For older eyes, the more protection against ultraviolet rays, the better. As it does with skin, UV creates free-radical damage that gradually affects your retinal cells. Protect yourself, especially during the brightest times of day (11 a.m. –3 p.m.), with large-framed sunglasses. Wraparound styles block out most light, limiting both vision damage and sun-induced wrinkles. Make sure the ones you buy not only look good but provide 100% UVA and UVB absorption, which gives the best protection against radiation reaching the eye and causing problems such as inflammation of the cornea or cataracts (see over for more on buying sunglasses).

Eat for healthy eyes

Your diet affects your eyes, too. As you age, toxins in the body cause your eyes to trade their bright, white color for something more yellow. (Start any detox and you'll notice how much clearer and more sparkling your eyes look.) You can eat for healthy eyes with carotene-rich foods. The most important carotenes are lutein, found in dark green leafy vegetables, and zeaxanthin, found in yellow and orange fruits and vegetables such as carrots, sweet potatoes, mangoes, and peaches. Dark purple foods like blueberries and blackberries also help strengthen your eyes, and vitamin-E-rich foods such as hazelnuts, almonds, and tomato paste are eye-friendly.

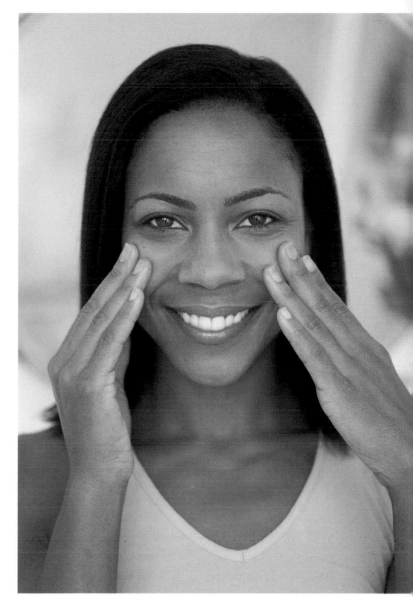

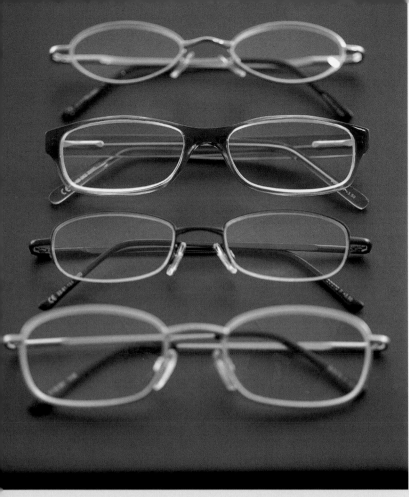

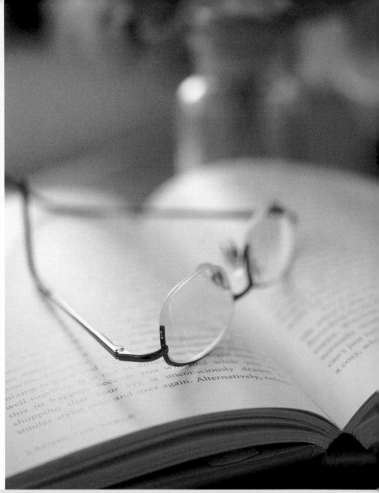

Help! I Need Glasses

Despite advances in contact lenses and even laser surgery, more than half of us with sight problems choose the glasses option. In fact, far from glasses being an eyesore, the right ones can actually be very flattering, helping to minimize your less-than-good points. Selecting the right frames takes time, so don't do it when you're rushing. And never shop for frames immediately after an eye test if you've had dilating eye drops, as you won't be able to see yourself properly!

How to choose the perfect frames

* Metal frames (usually made of titanium or stainless steel) suit most people and are a good first-time buy as they're discreet. Metal is also durable so should last for two to three years, by which time you'll be due another eye test and may possibly need a new pair.

* Rimless glasses are also a restrained first-time buy, but remember they are more fragile as the lens is unsupported, so treat them with care.
* The majority of other frames are made of plastic and are most flattering when toned with your hair. Black looks great with dark hair, and shades of tortoiseshell suit blonde to mid-brown hair.
* If you feel invisible behind glasses, try making a bolder statement with a heavier black or tortoiseshell style, which can look good even on smaller features.
* Make sure your eyes are in the middle of each frame and the top bar follows the line of your eyebrows.
* Your face shape determines which glasses will suit you. The most important rule is to avoid frames the same shape as your face. Long faces need frames that will counteract

length and narrowness, which means very small frames won't suit you. Instead choose medium- or larger-size frames with width to draw your face out at the sides. Square faces need to avoid anything too angular or hard, which will emphasize a strong jaw, and instead go for light, thin frames in a soft oval shape. Round faces should avoid soft, oval shapes and go for either square or horn-rimmed frames instead. Oval faces can wear anything including smaller frames, which can be unflattering on others, but bear in mind that the larger the frames, the more camouflage they provide for under-eye wrinkles and bags.

* Frames can also be used to distract from your least favorite feature. Horn-rimmed frames work well at drawing attention away from a double chin, and glasses with a lower bridge will shorten a long nose (as a higher bridge in a light color will lengthen a short one). You can also make close-set eyes seem wider apart by wearing small, lightweight frames with a narrow bridge.

Be savvy with sunglasses

Even on a cloudy day, up to 80% of UV light can reach your eyes, so sunglasses are much more than just a fashion accessory. Buy sunglasses offering 99–100% UV protection (look for confirmation on the swing tag). Glasses matching this standard can be found at all prices, so there's no need to buy designer unless you want to. Tints range from light to very dark; the lightest are only suitable for days when there's little sun, and very dark tints are needed for exceptionally sunny conditions such as skiing. Don't wear light-colored shades on anything but cloudy days, as they can actually allow more harmful rays to enter the eye on sunny days. The reason? They're dark enough to cause the pupil to dilate to compensate for the reduction in light, and by making the pupil dilate, they allow more harmful rays in. Style rules are the same as for prescription glasses, but it's worth remembering that the larger the frames, the more protection you'll get.

Far from glasses being an eyesore, the right ones can actually be very **flattering**, helping to minimize your less-than-good points. Take time to select the **right frames**.

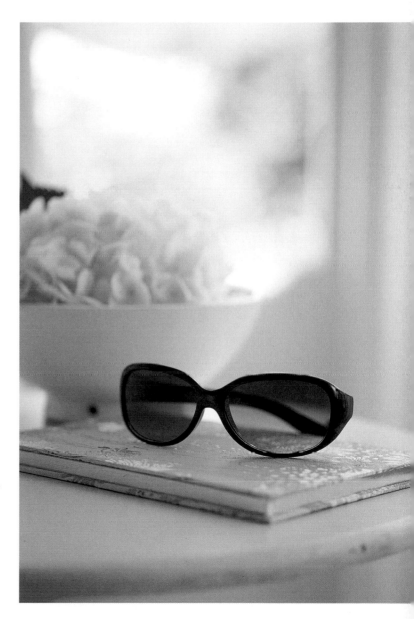

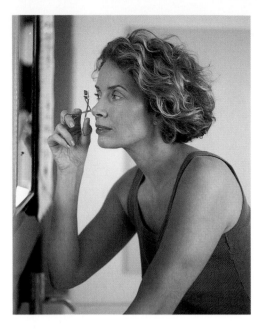

Makeup Tricks for Older Eyes

Makeup rules for glasses

Glasses do one of two things: they minimize your eyes, which means you need to enhance them (use eyeliner and curl your lashes before applying two coats of mascara); or they maximize everything behind the lens, which means makeup mistakes are on show (mascara clumps are particularly ugly, so avoid "body-building" types and go for a lengthening formula, which will have fewer fibers).

If your glasses are a bold color, don't try to compete with makeup. Instead, balance the effect with a well-defined, mid-toned mouth. Coloured-glass frames are also effective if your eyes are sensitive and run at the first sign of makeup. You can ditch the eyeliner and let your glasses do the talking.

Glasses and sunglasses will rub off foundation, especially around your nose. There's no way to avoid this, so spot-check occasionally and smooth things out with a quick blend.

Your brows (rather than the top rim of your glasses) should frame your face. Make them well defined by filling in with an eyeshadow one shade lighter than your brow hairs. Brush through with a clear mascara or an old toothbrush.

How to disguise aging eye shapes

Good eye makeup is all about creating an optical illusion, using dark colors to recede and light colors to accentuate. Here's how:

Deep-set eyes

You want to bring your eyes out, so use a light shade over your lids. Lining the top lash line from the center to the outer corner will also make your eyelashes look thicker, accentuating the eye rather than the recessive lid.

Droopy eyes

This is where clever shading comes in. To see the whole eye area, hold your mirror at a 45-degree angle below eye level and tilt your head back so the crease disappears. Now brush a light-colored eyeshadow over the lids and brow bone, and then apply a mid-tone shade in an arc over the entire crease area. Avoid using eyeliner and brush two coats of mascara through top and bottom lashes.

All eyes

A dot of cream shadow on the brow bone opens eyes up instantly, and another at the inside corner of the eyes next to the nose brightens the whites of your eyes. You can also use a white kohl pencil along the inside rim, but avoid brilliant whites (they look great in pictures, but not so good in real life). Cream or a slightly bluey white looks more natural.

Making up when you don't see so well

Don't avoid makeup for fear of making a mistake. Invest in a magnifying mirror, and carry a small one in your bag for on-the-spot checks. Make-up can be simple but still make a huge difference to your appearance. A compact cream-to-powder foundation is easy to use—just stroke the sponge over areas that need coverage—and cream eyeshadow and blusher are quick and simple to apply with fingers. Consider having your eyelashes dyed professionally (results last up to three months—the life of an eyelash), so all you need is a slick of clear mascara to define them. Strong shades of lipstick show up the slightest blip, so stick to more natural tones, and if lining your lips is tricky, choose a two-step (one colored, one clear), long-lasting lip product, which sets on your lips, eliminating the risk of "bleeding" into fine lines. The easiest option? Mistake-proof colored lip gloss—just apply to your bottom lip and smack lips together.

Lining the top **lash line** from the center to the outer corner will make eyelashes look **thicker**.

Lips: Plumping and Painting

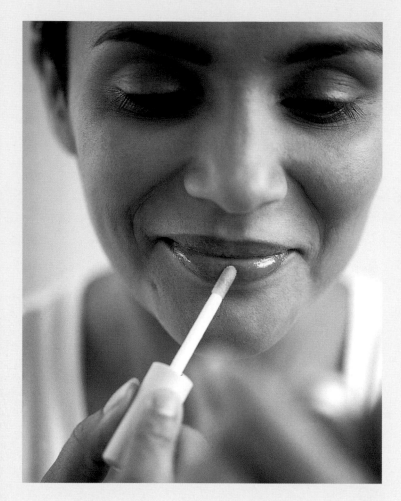

Some contain light-reflective pigments to literally bounce light away and create the illusion of a fuller mouth. Others contain a mildly irritating ingredient like chili, clove oil, or cinnamon extract which, when applied to the lips, causes them to tingle. This irritation also makes the tissues swell slightly and, violà, you have lips that look fuller instantly. Once you get used to the sensation, the second type gives more significant results. Another way to irritate your lips mildly so they swell slightly is to buff them gently using an old toothbrush, followed by a generous slick of lip balm.

Painting

* The right lipstick can do wonders for less-than-luscious lips, and can also take years off you. If you don't care to try the testers in your local store to see what suits you (and who does?), hold them up to your lips and you'll see right away which ones brighten up your skin tone.
* Dark colors make lips recede, while lighter ones make them stand out. This means avoiding matte, opaque darker lipsticks, which will make your lips look thinner, and choosing light to medium colors in moisturizing formulas (but avoid frosted shades, which just draw attention to fine lines).
* Loss of a strong outline around your lips means you need to add it in yourself. To make lips stand out and strengthen a weak lip line, use a fine brush to draw a line of concealer around your whole lip area before blending the edges away. Or use a lip pencil in a neutral shade just outside your natural lip line, but make sure it meets your own lip line perfectly at the corners of your mouth. And always choose a neutral shade for when your lipstick fades, as you don't want to be left with an unnatural line around your mouth (like an aging Hollywood star).
* Makeup artists apply foundation over the lips before painting on color to ensure lasting-power. Another way to create an undercoat is to fill in your lips with lipliner, which gives lipstick something to grab hold of. This is also a good idea if you're wearing gloss, as it provides a base to stop the gloss from sliding off too quickly.

Young lips are plump and rosy, but age causes a loss of volume and color, plus fullness around the outline, which is why lipstick can "bleed" into fine lines around your mouth.

Plumping

One way to deal with the deflation is a cosmetic filler (see page 27), but don't overdo it—celebrity magazines are full of mouths that don't fit the face they belong to! Luckily, there are plenty of other ways to make your lips look larger without resorting to needles.

Lip-plumping products work in one of two ways. All will moisturize deeply while providing a very flattering high gloss.

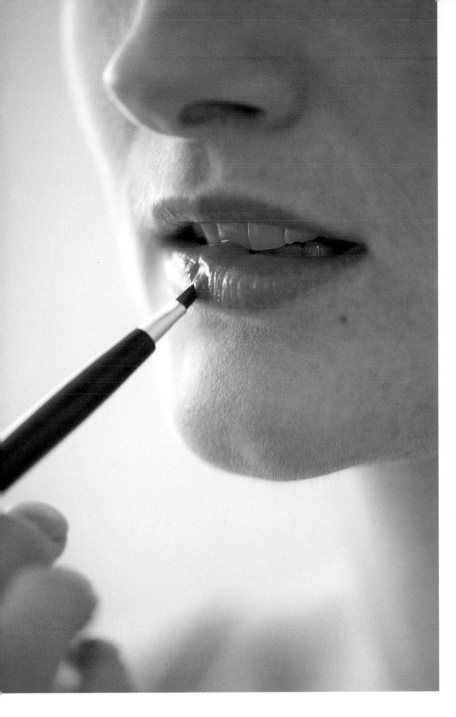

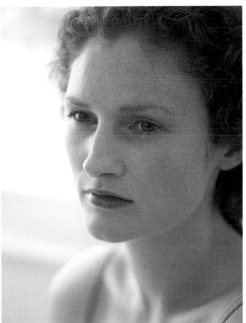

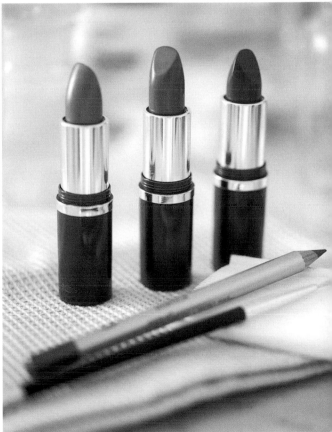

* Lip gloss reflects light, making lips look fuller, but go easy on the application as gloss will "bleed" easier than lipstick. A better idea is to apply your usual lipstick and then highlight the center of your lips with a dab of gloss to catch the light and magnify your mouth.

* Make your upper lip stand out by applying a dab of highlighter just above your Cupid's bow. Alternatively, use a white eye pencil drawn lightly above the Cupid's bow, but apply it very sparingly and blend away any hard edges.

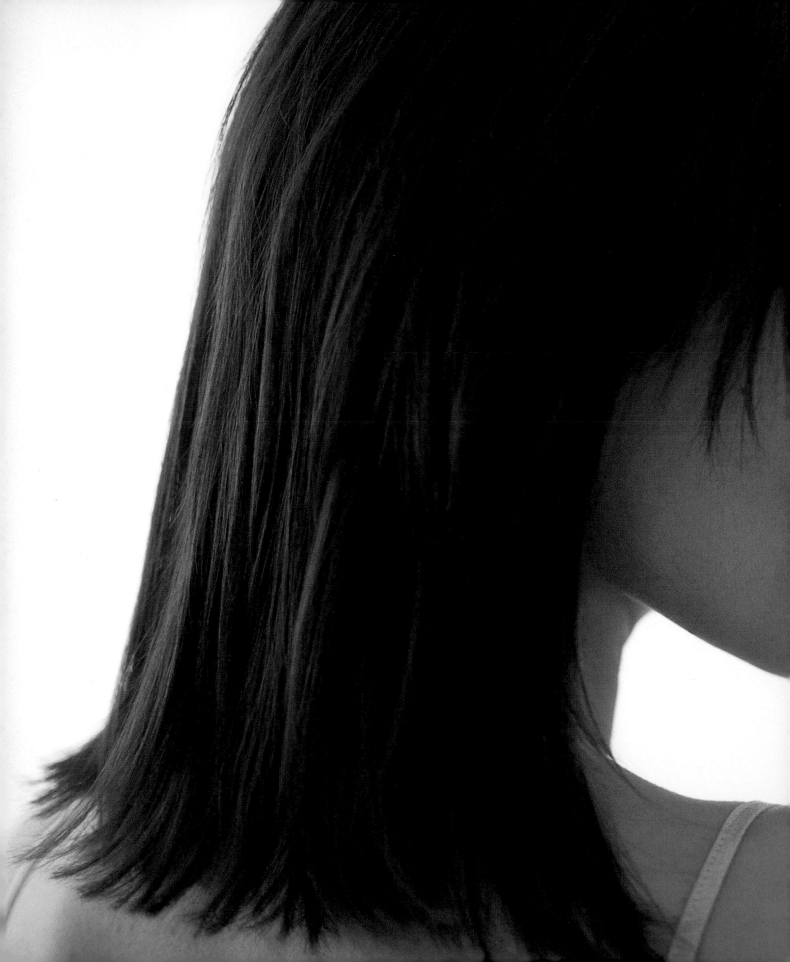

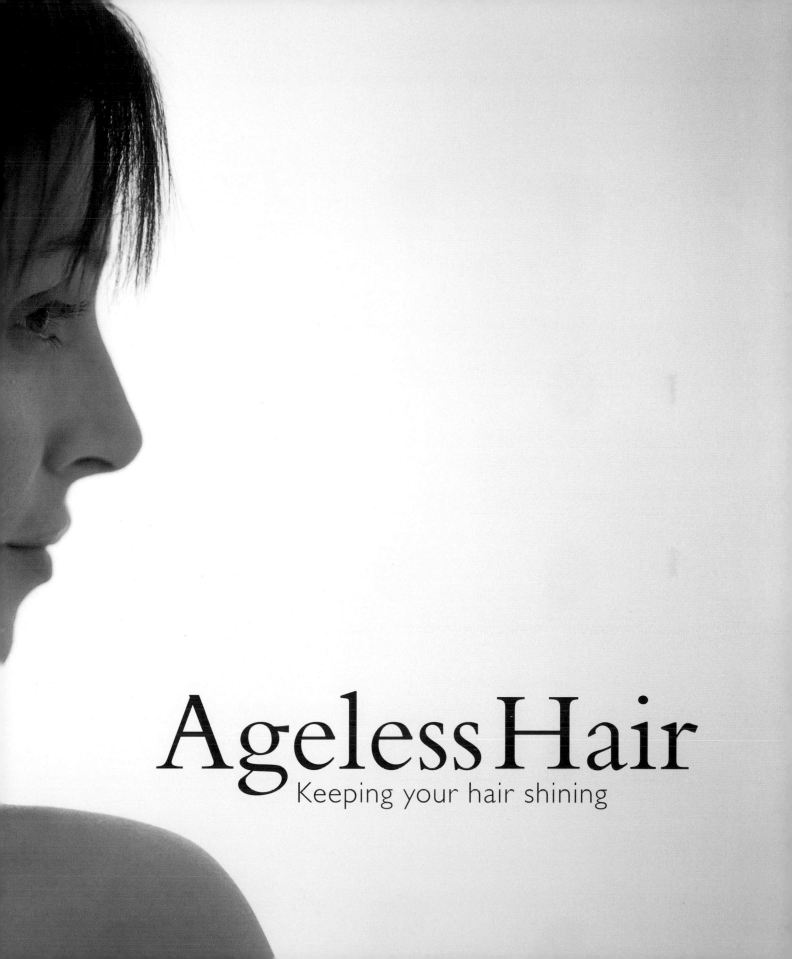

Ageless Hair
Keeping your hair shining

Age-defying Hair Styling Tips

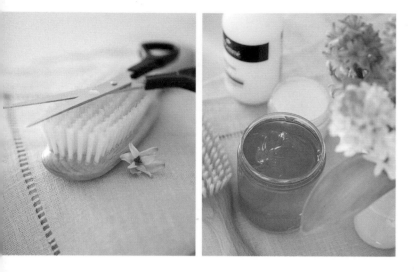

The right hairstyle can take years off you—or put years on. Top hairdressers Steven Goldsworthy and Paul Matthews (see Directory) help you get it right.

Steven Goldsworthy

* You don't wear the same clothes you did 20 years ago, so why the same hair? Keeping the style of your youth can be very aging. (Think Liza Minnelli and Donatella Versace.)
* After a certain age, wearing your hair forward is a bad idea, as nature has already started to drag down your features without your hair helping it along. Much better is to wear hair back, which will take your face with it.
* Avoid a bob that stops at your chin, as this will emphasize any developing jowls. Instead, choose a cut that finishes either above or below your jawline.
* Unless you have elfin features that look swamped with too much hair, leave hair longer at the back to soften your jaw.
* A soft, layered style that frames your face is very flattering. Keep hair flatter around your ears and ensure you have width at your temples to accentuate cheekbones (and counteract that "maturing" jaw).
* When you notice your jaw looking heavier it's time for a shorter style, as long hair will drag your face down. And never, ever, have hair that reaches past your elbows.

* Talk (and listen!) to your stylist, who can take into account everything from your dress sense to the amount of time you spend on your hair.
* Gray hair is coarser, so invest in a serum, which works by coating the outer layer to make your hair look smoother. It also works like a rain hat, protecting your hair from frizziness in damp weather. And look out for shampoos and conditioners formulated for coarse hair, or labeled "deep conditioning" or "moisturizing."
* Cutting techniques like texturizing and point-cutting can help control coarser hair. Ask your hairdresser for advice.

Paul Matthews

* Whatever age you are, it's still about what suits your face shape. Following high-fashion trends looks like you're trying too hard. Most older fashion icons have well-groomed hair in a classic style rather than the latest look. Great examples of this are Madonna, Lulu, and Sharon Osbourne.
* Take pictures of favorite styles to show your hairdresser (it can be part of a hairstyle, such as the bangs, rather than the whole look). Be aware that pictures in magazines are heavily styled and the cut may actually be very simple. The less styled your chosen picture, the better chance you'll have of achieving the same look at home.
* Some people dress up to visit a salon, but wearing your usual clothes allows a stylist to get a true picture of you.
* The most unflattering style for an older woman is long hair with a middle parting. If you like long hair, part it on the side and make sure you have softness around your face.
* Wearing your hair back gives the impression of lifting your face, but anything too tight looks harsh and also puts pressure on your front hairline.
* Visit your hairdresser regularly. Mussy, undressed hair may look good in your 20s, but won't look so good in your 40s.
* Don't over-style your hair with too much hairspray; "stuck" hair is very aging. Better choices are gel or mousse, which give more texture and shine. Avoid trying to make your hair look too perfect or done—a big age giveaway.

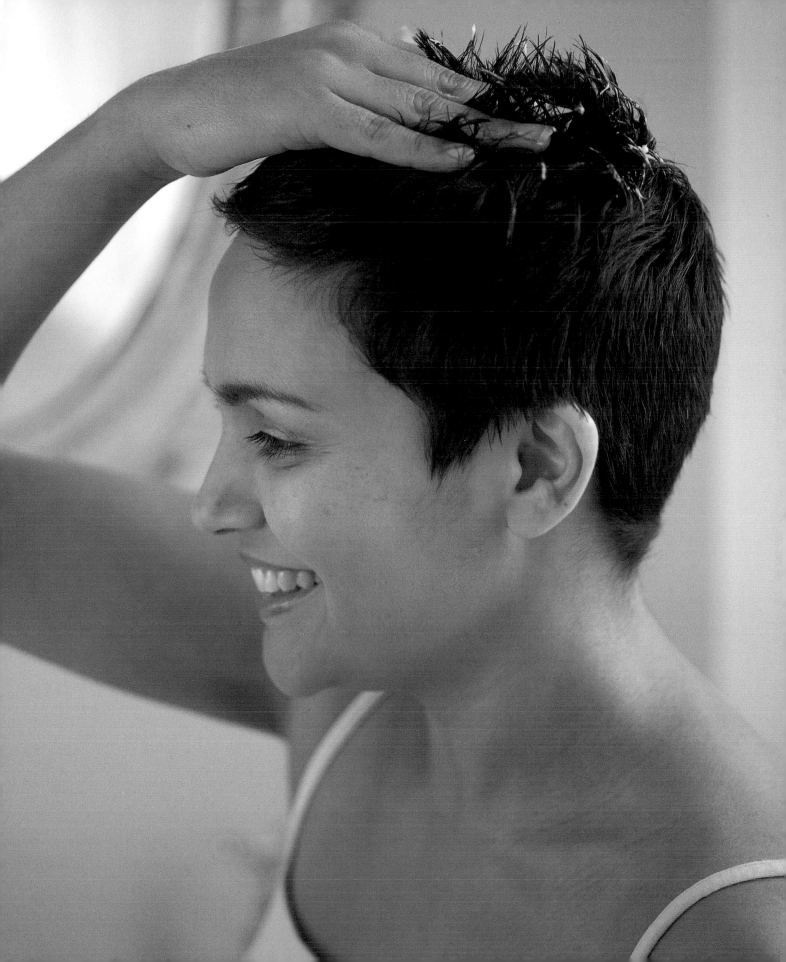

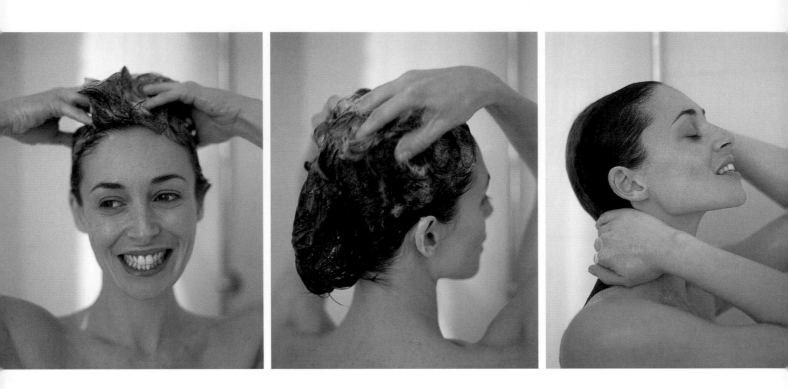

Thinning Hair: the Causes and the Cures

Thinning hair is not just a male problem. Glenn Lyons, Clinical Director at Philip Kingsley and Fellow at The Institute of Trichologists (see Directory), believes that thinning hair is becoming more common in women. But there's no need to panic if your hair looks less plentiful than it used to, as there's a cure for many common causes of hair loss.

Genetic hair loss

This occurs in women who have genetically predisposed hair follicles that gradually become sensitive to normal levels of male hormones in the body. The hair follicles will become increasingly finer until eventually growth stops altogether. This type of hair loss mostly affects the top area of the scalp and happens over a number of years rather than months. If you notice your hair getting finer but no extra hairs are clogging the shower plughole, you should visit a trichologist for a diagnosis. And don't hold off until the problem becomes very noticeable, as genetic hair loss is totally preventable, but only

partially reversible. In Glenn's opinion, the best treatment is topical hormones applied to the affected area at night (available from selected trichological clinics—see Directory).

Increased shedding

There are many reasons why you may be finding more hair on your clothes or in the plughole, but Glenn believes that in normal healthy women the most important things to ensure are adequate amounts of iron (ferritin) and vitamin B12. Ask your doctor for a blood test; results should be at least mid-range (if in doubt, take your result to a trichologist). Hair shedding is often self-correcting, but if the amount of hair coming out continues past six to eight weeks, visit a trichologist. Hair can be a great barometer of health, which means everything from a course of antibiotics to poor diet can affect it, and in most cases the hair you're losing today will have been caused by something that started three months ago. Glenn recommends a good balance of protein and carbohydrates (forget your Atkins diet) and never going more than four hours without eating. Hair follicles are one of the fastest-growing cells in the body so need a lot of energy, but as hair is low in your body's priority list (losing your hair isn't life-threatening, after all), not giving yourself enough nutrients means your hair is one of the first things to suffer.

Post-partum hair loss

It's estimated that around 50% of new mothers suffer hair loss, some more dramatically than others. The reason for this is simple. When you become pregnant, a surge of female hormones means more hair is retained on your head (usually 10% of our hair is in its "falling" stage), and most women say their hair has more volume during pregnancy. But once your baby is born, your hormones start returning to normal and the hair you would have lost naturally over the last nine months starts falling out (in a far shorter space of time!). This is absolutely temporary and self-correcting, so although a little unsettling, it's really nothing to worry about.

In most cases your hair should return to normal after two to three months (recovery time can be delayed due to breast-feeding), but if there's no improvement after this time, the best advice is to visit a trichologist, as your hair loss could be due to other reasons.

Aggressive styling

There's no doubt about it. Certain hairdressing techniques can damage your hair, causing breakage that looks like hair loss. An easy way to tell the difference is to feel the roots of your hair (spiky broken ends will feel very different to hair shedding from the roots). Whether it's a hot hairdryer held too close to your hair, brushing your hair when it's wet, or pulling out Velcro rollers too harshly, aggressive handling and heat both evaporate your hair's moisture levels. Styling your hair is fine; just do it gently. Swap your bristle brush for one with widely spaced plastic prongs or a wide-tooth comb, and use a good "moisturizing" conditioner, which will help your hair retain elasticity and moisture levels.

Styling your hair is fine; just do it **gently**. Swap your bristle brush for one with widely spaced plastic prongs or a **wide-tooth comb**, and use a good "moisturizing" conditioner.

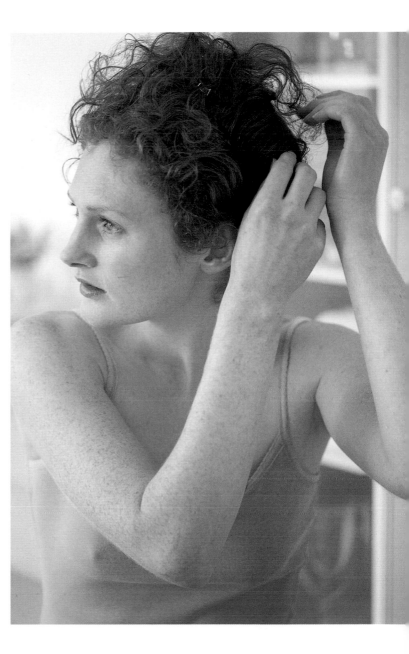

How to Look Like you've got Twice as Much Hair

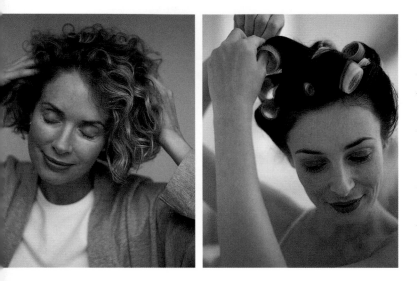

1 Forget the rule about shorter styles being best for fine hair. In fact, short layers are very aging—just think of your grandmother's shampoo and set! Far more modern is a shoulder-length bob with long layers to give volume and shape. And you can still put it up, too.

2 Ask your hairdresser for cutting techniques that give your hair volume. Point-cutting, slicing, tapering, and razoring all take weight out of the hair so it doesn't hang flat.

3 A good volumizing or thickening shampoo can work like a collagen injection for the hair. Ask your stylist what they recommend. Far from being commission-hungry, your hairdresser actually knows your hair better than anyone. And don't be put off by the price—you usually get what you pay for. Lastly, consider investing in a styling spray from the same range. Products are formulated to work together, so it's worth sticking with one brand.

4 Wash fine hair daily if possible, as it goes limp quicker than any other hair type. But use conditioner sparingly, just on the mid-lengths and ends, or your hair could dry flatter than it was before.

5 For a body-building blow-dry, hang your head upside down to blast volume into the roots. Or, even better, dry hair in the opposite direction to how your hair grows, which means raking all your hair over to one side, and then switching hands and raking it over to the other. Keep alternating until your hair is nearly dry, then swap your fingers for a plastic pronged brush and smooth the surface.

6 Teasing hair may sound 1950s, but done gently it can hold your newly styled volume in place without any damage. Take a section of hair and, holding it without tension, use a wide-tooth comb to tease the roots. To remove tangles after your night out, start combing through the ends and work up.

7 If you only have a minute, hang your head upside down and massage your roots. Spray with a styling or fixing spray and, voilà, big hair!

8 Velcro rollers are much kinder than heated ones, but only use on short to medium-length hair, as longer hair will tangle. When choosing your roller size, remember that hair needs to go around a roller at least one and a half times to hold it in place. You can put Velcro rollers in damp hair and wait for it to dry, or for quicker results in just-styled warm hair (when the hair cools, it will "set" the style). Or, for between-shampoos styling, put the rollers in dry hair, heat them with a hairdryer for five minutes, wait until they've cooled right down, and then unwind gently. For extra oomph, hang your head upside down and spray with a fixing product before raking hair through with your fingers.

9 Velvet-coated heated rollers are the best bet for long hair. If the result is too curly, only leave them in for half the recommended time. This cuts down on heat damage, too.

10 For a quick-fix plumper, gently rub sections of hair between your fingers and thumb. This will fluff up the cuticles, creating instant volume.

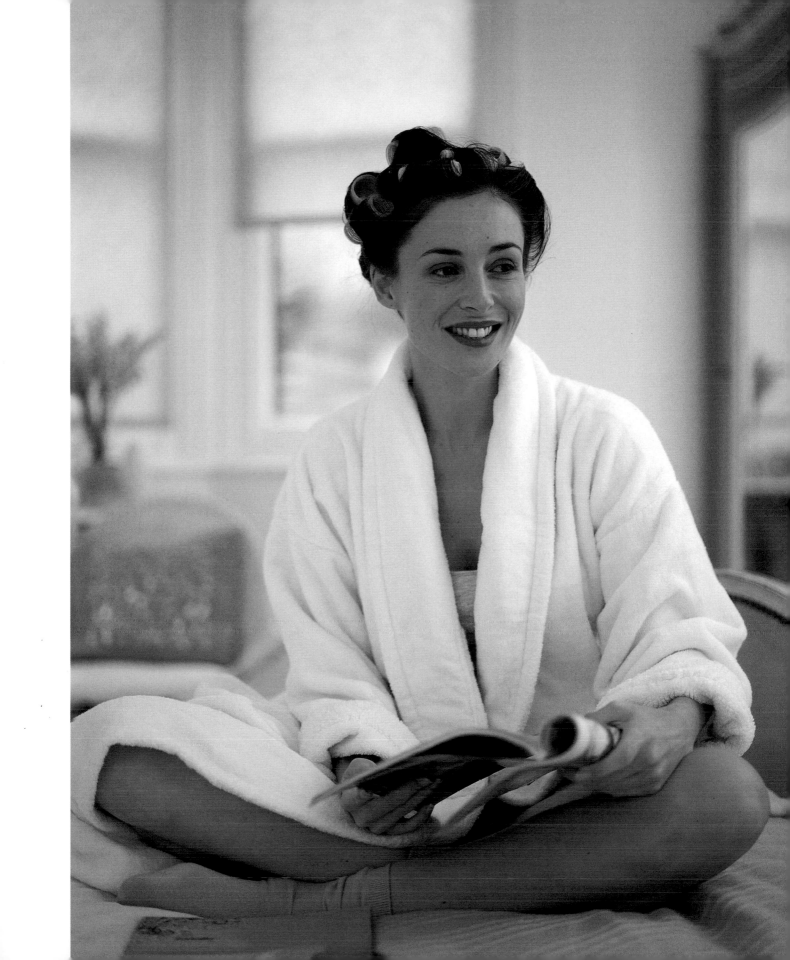

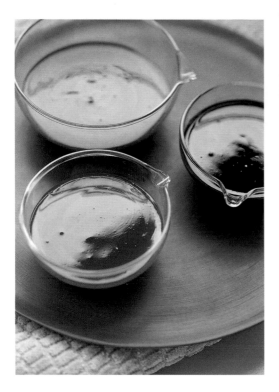

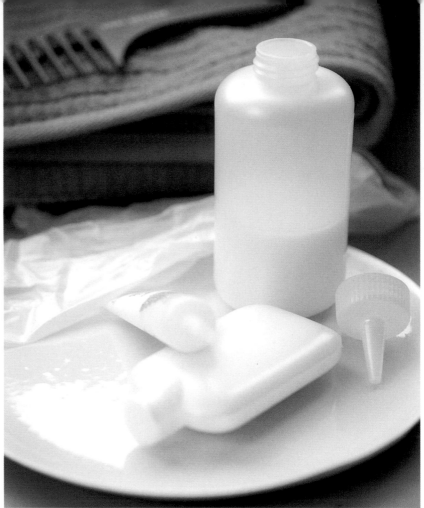

Coloring: How to Get it Right

How soon you go gray depends upon your genes, but many of us are now going gray sooner, due partly to our stressful lives. An unlucky few may spot their first gray hair at 20, and 50% of women will be gray by the age of 50. But look upon coloring as a chance to improve on nature, and suddenly those first gray hairs won't seem so bad after all.

According to Steven Goldsworthy, skin tone changes as we age and our hair starts to turn gray. This means that if you try to keep the hair color you had at 20, chances are you'll end up looking sallow-skinned, plus darker hair also emphasizes lines, making your skin look older.

Steven recommends lifting your hair a couple of shades lighter. The best way to do this while hiding the first signs of gray is with highlights or lowlights, which can work like a

mini facelift. For best results these need to be done professionally, but if salon prices are out of your range, ask your hairdresser about trainee nights, where a fully qualified stylist will oversee your color every step of the way. Or call your local higher education college and ask if they run a hairdressing course. All trainee hairdressers need to practice on real people, and are never let loose on anyone until they know what they're doing.

Your other option is an overall color, which will give your hair more shine than high- or lowlights. Paul Matthews advises using semi-permanent colorants, which are a great way to color your whole head without that unnatural "block" effect you can get with permanent dyes. In fact, Paul advises avoiding permanent colorants for as long as you can get

Warm **semi-permanent** shades will give your hair a shiny, youthful glow and can last between 6 and 24 shampoos (read the box), covering **40–50% gray**.

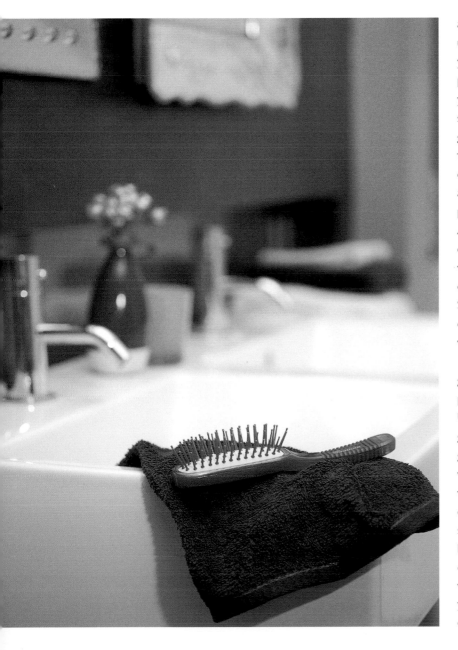

away with it (until you are 80% gray and upward), as they contain more chemicals and you're also stuck with the result. Warm semi-permanent shades will give your hair a shiny, youthful glow and can last between 6 and 24 shampoos (read the box), covering 40–50% gray. Remember, if you have to mix two bottles together (or twist a bottle to mix its two compartments), then chemicals are involved and the color inside is either a long-lasting semi-permanent (up to 24 washes) or permanent. And, while older women look best with hair a couple of shades lighter than their natural color, very light blonde hair is also aging as it washes out skin tone (and also doesn't cover gray well). So if you've been using peroxide until now, consider swapping to a honey-blonde tone, which will be far more flattering.

And think twice before deciding to grow gray gracefully as gray hair can drain your face, plus it absorbs the light, making hair look dull. Unfortunately, women who look good with gray hair tend to be the ones who would look good whatever their hair color! Your skin tone will also determine if you should stick with what nature intended. Either dark or pale complexions look best with gray hair, with sallow skins and redheads rarely finding silver hair flattering. If you do decide to go gray, more colorful makeup is essential to avoid looking washed out, and if your gray starts turning yellow use a purple- or blue-based shampoo or conditioner to neutralize the tone.

Coloring your Hair at Home

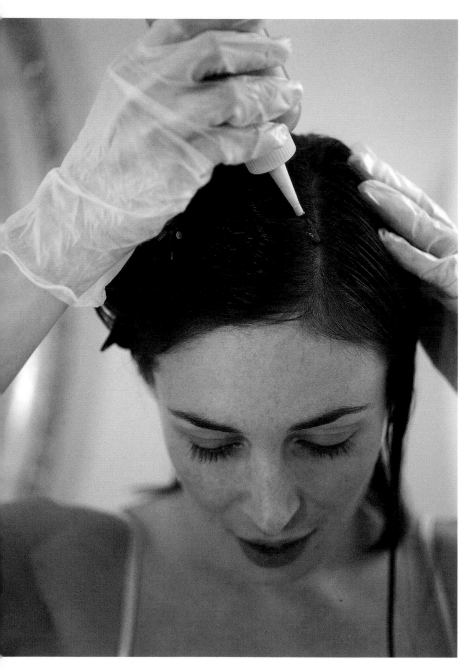

What most hairdressers probably won't tell you is that home and salon colorants are virtually identical, so what you're paying for at a salon is both the ease and the expertise.

What can I use?

The array of products on the home-coloring shelves is baffling at best, so here's a simple guide to what's available.

Up to 20% gray

A semi-permanent color similar to your natural shade will blend a few gray hairs in with the rest. These contain no chemicals, so they coat rather than penetrate your hair. They last between six and eight shampoos, but longer if your hair is "porous" (damaged). That's because when hair is damaged the cuticle's not flat against the shaft, allowing more color to get inside.

Up to 50% gray

Time to step up to a longer-lasting semi-permanent (once called demi-permanent), which contains a small amount of hydrogen peroxide, but no ammonia. This penetrates a little but not as much as a permanent, giving results that last up to 24 washes.

Over 80% gray

The only way to cover this much color is with a permanent dye, which will penetrate the hair shaft. If in doubt, choose a lighter rather than darker shade, which will be easier to color over should you dislike the result.

Work the colorant into your hair, not your scalp.
To touch up permanent color, just apply to roots.

Troubleshooting tips

* If you're not sure about what to use, phone one of the advisory services (find the number on most colorant boxes). Trained staff can answer questions on any make of color and they'll even do a strand test if you send them a cutting of your hair.
* Always do a skin test each time you color your hair (follow instructions in the pack). And wait 48 hours before you go ahead (this is the time it takes between contact with the allergen and any potential reaction), to allow any sensitivity to show up. If you do react, don't use the color or any other product. Instead, call the company helpline (on the box) for advice. This may involve diagnostic patch testing by a dermatologist to confirm the cause of your reaction. You can then avoid it in future by checking ingredients on the box before buying.
* The ingredient most commonly associated with allergic reactions is the hair dye paraphenylene diamine (PPD), and unfortunately this is present in all permanent hair colors. Allergies can be serious enough to warrant medical attention (and occasionally even fatal). Once you've been diagnosed, using a temporary, wash-out color or high- or lowlights are your only options.
* If you're allergic (or sensitive) to another chemical in traditional hair dyes, you can try one of the new herbal-based permanent hair colors (see Directory). By adding plant-based ingredients, including anti-inflammatories, and removing paraben preservatives and resorcinol, these formulations minimize the likelihood of chemical problems such as scalp sensitivity.
* Less important for your health, but vital for your hair, is a strand test. Do this at the same time as your skin test and you'll only have to mix the ingredients once. Not only will you discover the final color result (keep an eye on the time so you know exactly how long to leave it on), but also how the colorant will affect the condition of your hair.
* If you're unhappy with a semi-permanent result, frequent washing with an anti-dandruff or "clarifying" shampoo will

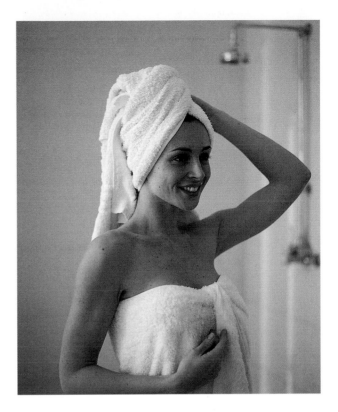

fade it faster. Never try to rectify a permanent color mistake yourself, or you will make matters worse. Instead, swallow your pride, cover your hair with a hat, and go to a salon for professional advice. And don't worry: they've seen it all before—and worse!

At-home coloring techniques

* Take off any rings that could tear the plastic gloves, wear old clothes and an even older towel around your shoulders, and if you're using a permanent color splatter-proof your bathroom, too.
* Wipe the skin around your hairline (and ears) with petroleum jelly to avoid staining, and use a timer to ensure your timing is exact (most home-coloring disasters are caused by leaving it on too long).
* Work the colorant into your hair, not your scalp. And, for touch-up applications of permanent color, just apply to your roots or you'll suffer stripes where your hair has become overloaded. Then just work it through the rest of your hair for a few minutes at the end.
* A few gray hairs around your hairline? Mascara in a shade close to your own, applied from root to tip, will do a great job of disguising them until your next coloring session.

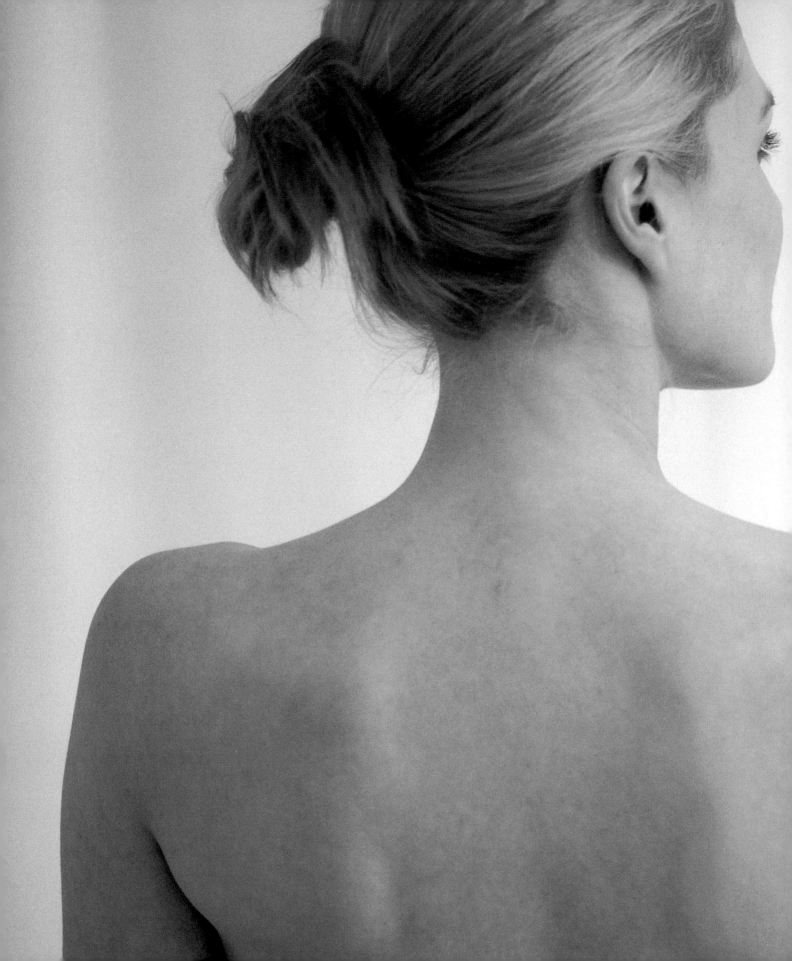

AgelessBody

Keeping your body beautiful

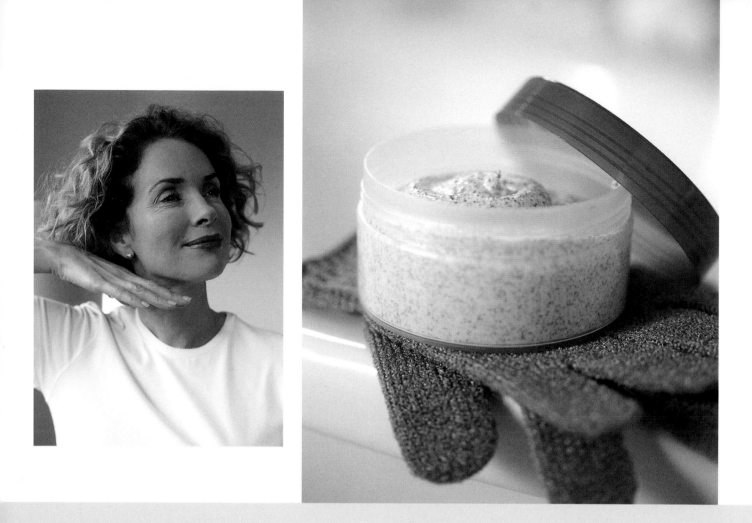

Holding Back the Years: Dimples and Wrinkles

Neck

The skin on your neck is paler, thinner, and drier than the rest of your body, so is likely to look crepey more quickly, too. The first rule of neck care is to treat it like an extension of your face, so whether you're exfoliating, moisturizing, or cleansing, extend the products south. The way you apply is important, too—upward strokes with the back of your hand are perfect, as palm pressure can be too forceful. Foundation shouldn't stop at your jaw either, but you only need a little as skin tone will be more even on your neck, so use the residue left on your hand, sponge, or foundation brush. And never skip sunscreen on your neck, as the pale skin here is more likely to burn. Lastly, practice perfect posture (see over) to guard against the dreaded turkey neck. Holding your head high and

your shoulders back will not only strengthen your neck's supporting muscles to prevent creasing, but also help smooth away wrinkles already there.

Bust and décolletage

If you're the proud owner of a medium to large bust, you'll be carrying between three and five pounds of weight, which (not surprisingly) can stretch your skin, making it look looser. Wearing a good supportive bra will help maintain skin tone, so get yourself measured for free at your local department store. And buy a good sports bra for exercising, as this is when your bust needs help the most. Using a firming cream can stimulate collagen to keep the area looking younger and go some way to reverse past damage. Use your opposite

Use **sweeping strokes** on dry skin in the direction of your heart to stimulate not just your skin but the **lymph** nodes underneath.

hand to stroke firmly upward toward your shoulder, so you don't drag skin down. Your décolletage is also where sun damage shows up fast as it's so often exposed to the environment (without the protection you give your face), so extend your sunscreen downwards during summer. Need inspiration to do the housework? Washing windows is a great bust-firming exercise—the larger and more energetic the movements, the better!

Bottom

An oatmeal-like bottom can be much improved by brushing your skin to boost circulation. Before your bath or shower, use sweeping strokes on dry skin in the direction of your heart to stimulate not just your skin but the lymph nodes underneath. Massage can also help break down and disperse the fatty cells below your skin's surface, and you can make your own anti-cellulite oil with two teaspoons of carrier oil, plus two drops of cypress essential oil (to stimulate) and two drops of juniper essential oil (a diuretic). Smooth on daily and then gently pinch and roll your cellulite dimples between fingers and thumb.

Not surprisingly, any form of cardiovascular exercise will boost circulation while burning fat. For best results, choose activities that target your legs and bottom, such as cycling, fast walking, and running. Lastly, eat a diet rich in antioxidants and vitamin C (that means at least five portions of fresh fruit and veg a day), which will strengthen the collagen fibers in your skin responsible for elasticity (meaning that lumps and bumps will be less noticeable below the surface). Cut down on foods high in fat, salt, and sugar, and drink eight glasses of metabolism-boosting water a day, as dehydration is a major cause of sluggish circulation.

Legs

Standing for long periods makes any legs vulnerable to varicose veins, which form when the veins in your legs can't return blood to your heart efficiently, causing it to stagnate and your veins to swell. Your best defense is regular exercise, especially walking, and increasing the circulation in your legs while sitting by stretching them out in front of you and pointing and flexing your feet five times. And, while surgical stockings are a known deterrent, Lycra fashion stockings may also help control the problem.

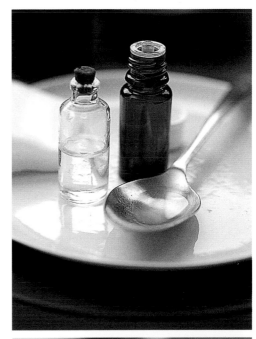

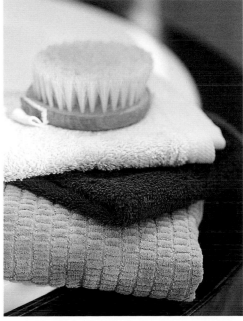

Straight Talking

If you want to take years off your looks instantly, there are few better ways than simply standing taller. Walking like an old person, with hunched shoulders, not only causes back pain but can make you look lazy, frumpy, and lacking in confidence (how you hold yourself is one of the first things people notice about you).

Your head weighs around 11 lbs (5 kg), so by hanging it forward you're putting a massive strain on your back and spine. Over time this will weaken neck muscles, making your shoulders even more rounded. Bad posture has also been linked to arthritis, digestive disorders, repetitive strain injury, and sciatica, but the benefits of good posture are instant. You can add two inches to your height (we start to shrink from the age of 40, so need all the help we can get!) and look up to 6½ lb (3 kg) lighter, just by standing tall. Rounded shoulders also reduce your bust by a cup size, but standing with your shoulders drawn back will make them look twice as perky.

Carrying yourself like a sack of potatoes is simply a habit, and one you can break with practice. And it's worth it. Walk like a taller, thinner, younger person, and that's exactly what you'll look like.

Perfect posture

Good posture begins at ground level, as the position of your feet directly affects the alignment of your hips and spine. Inward rolling of the feet is a problem for many of us, giving the whole body a slouched, curled-over appearance. Get your feet well aligned and your whole body posture will improve. Try this exercise:

1 Stand with knees soft and feet facing forward, hip width apart. Ensure your weight is in the center of your feet by rolling forward and back until you find the middle position.
2 Tighten your buttock muscles and draw in your stomach as if trying to touch your spine with your tummy button.
3 Stretch your spine up, drawing your shoulder blades together without lifting your shoulders.
4 Lastly, imagine you're a puppet being pulled up by a string attached to the crown of your head. Relax your jaw and drop your shoulders.
5 As you move around, the aim is to have your ears, thighs, and insteps in line, and while sitting, your shoulders should be balanced over your hips so you don't slump.

Five-second fix: We all walk taller when we're happy, so remind yourself of something cheerful as you leave the house and you'll stride out with your head held high.

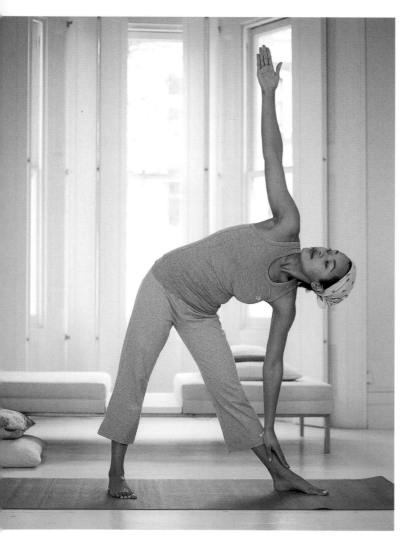

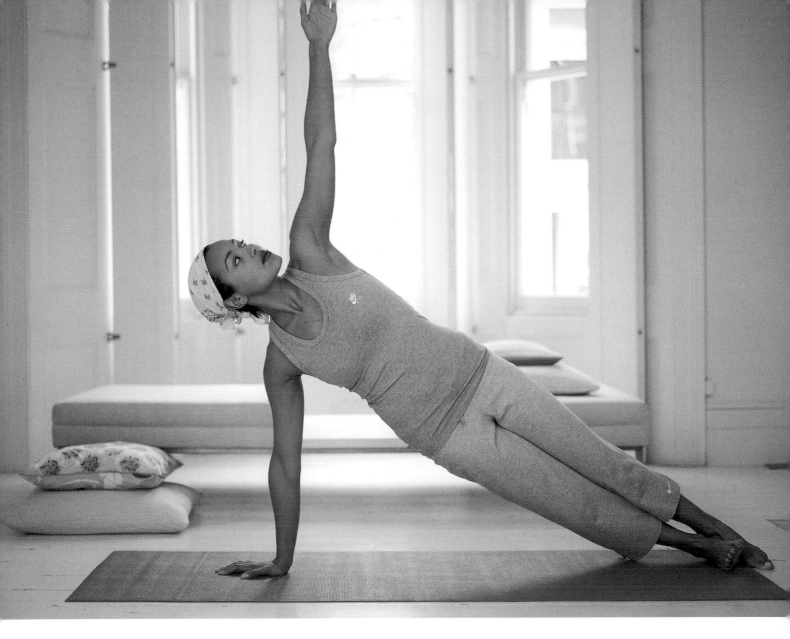

Exercises for better posture

★ Your spine's support system is the transversus abdominis muscle, which wraps around your middle and is weak in bad back sufferers. The best moves to strengthen this muscle are done slowly and gently. Yoga, Pilates, t'ai chi, and Feldenkrais will all improve your posture while alleviating the back problems that over 40% of us suffer each year.

★ Regularly contracting your pelvic floor muscles will improve your posture considerably. Squeeze as if you're trying to stop yourself going to the toilet, while consciously tightening your abdominals.

★ Try this Pilates move known as "Zip Up and Hollow" (it's also said to be great for your sex life). Sit upright on a chair, take a deep breath in, and as you breathe out draw up the muscles of your pelvic floor, again as if you're trying to stop yourself peeing. Think of drawing them together from side to side rather than from bottom to top—and then lift up a little. It may help to imagine you're doing up an internal zipper from your pelvic floor, while you hollow your lower abdominals back towards your spine. Breathe in and release.

Dump your Toxic Overload

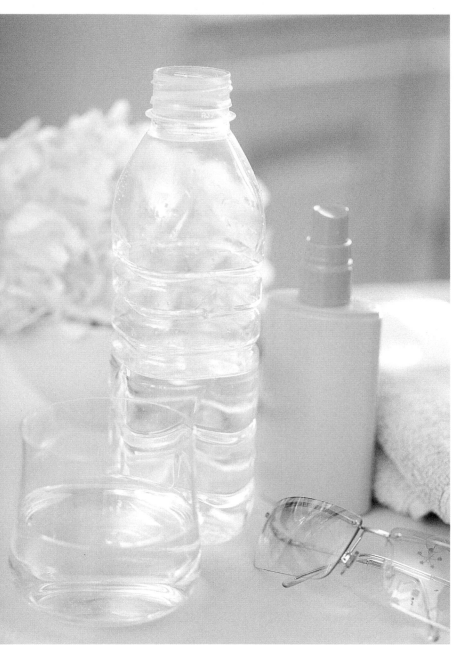

It's estimated that 70,000 chemicals foreign to the human body are in common use today. And if that wasn't enough, another 1,000 are being introduced each year. Our bodies are being contaminated by substances that have never been a part of the environment before, and the more toxins you have in your body, the more you will struggle to look and feel good.

Toxins are everywhere. In the air we breathe, sprayed over the food we eat, in the chemicals we use to clean our homes, and in the beauty products we buy. This accumulation of toxins has been blamed for many current health issues, from a rise in infertility to the food intolerances and allergies so common today. And these same toxins are also very bad news for your skin, as they create free radicals (see page 16), which damage healthy cell renewal, causing skin to age more quickly.

We may not be able to choose the air we breathe, but we can make other choices to lessen our toxic exposure.

How to lessen the load

★ Avoid chemicals in food, such as artificial colorings and flavorings in convenience foods and already-prepared meals and desserts, and artificial flavorings and additives such as monosodium glutamate. Organic food, which contains fewer pesticides, is your best choice.

★ Consider switching your usual cleaning products to environmentally safer ones, which are now widely available at all supermarkets and health-food stores.

Fill up on antioxidant foods, use skincare containing antioxidants, and drink **eight glasses** of water a day.

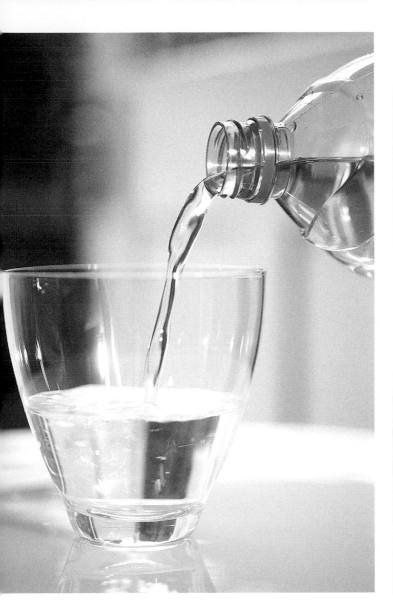

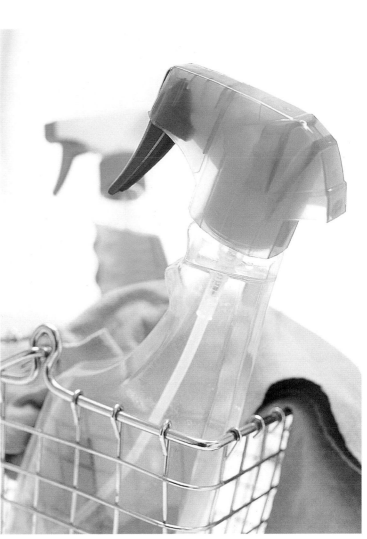

* Reduce your exposure to radiation by ditching your microwave oven, minimizing your cell phone usage, and limiting the time you spend in front of a computer or TV.

* The majority of beauty products contain chemical colorants and preservatives. Read the labels and cut back on products containing parabens, sodium lauryl or laureth sulphate, synthetic fragrances and colorants, petrochemicals, and PABA sunscreens. Or choose from a range that promises to be 100% natural (see Directory).

* The thinning of the ozone layer caused by air pollution means the sun's ultraviolet rays are now less filtered, and therefore more dangerous. The most common form of skin cancer now affects 800,000 Americans a year. The majority of sunscreens contain chemicals that are absorbed into the skin, adding to your toxic overload. Far better are non-chemical sunscreens, which contain minerals (titanium dioxide or zinc oxide) that sit on the skin's surface (see Directory).

* Limit your exposure to pollutants by avoiding walking (and never exercising) by a busy road. Stay out of smoke-filled rooms, and surround yourself with plants that filter out indoor pollution.

* Fight back by filling up on antioxidant foods (see over), using skincare products containing antioxidants (see page 16), and drinking at least eight glasses of pure water a day to give yourself an internal wash.

The most **anti-aging foods** you can eat are the ones that help mop up **free radicals** in your body. It's no surprise that they're mostly **fresh** fruit and vegetables.

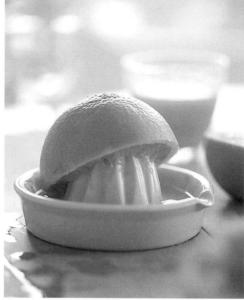

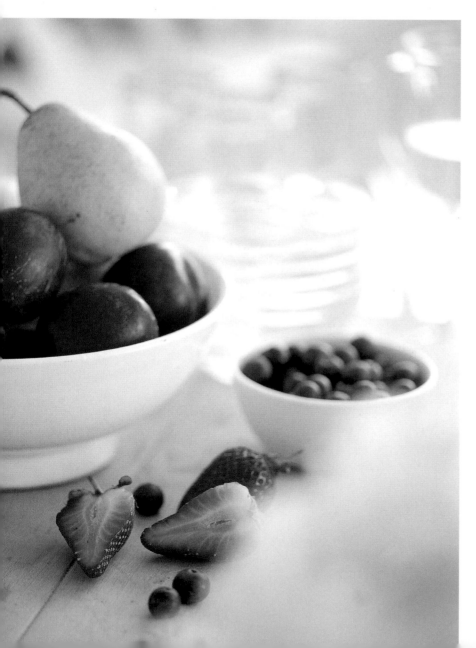

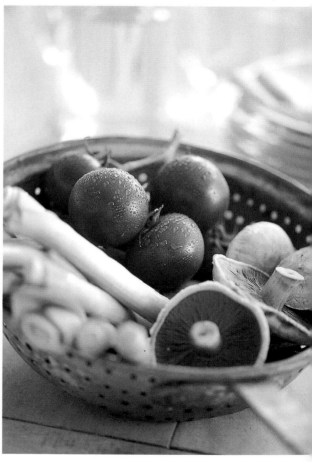

Stay Younger Longer Diet

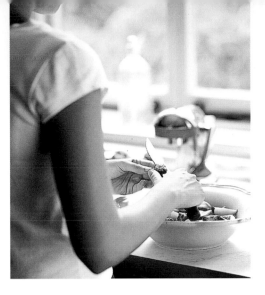

There's no doubt that eating a nutrient-packed diet is the easiest way to live a long, healthy life. The average woman in the United States lives to 79 years, but experts believe you can extend this by an impressive 10–15 years with the right nutrition. Luckily this doesn't mean avoiding jelly doughnuts forever. Food is one of life's pleasures, and not giving yourself treats would be a real shame. So if you've had a "bad" day, don't worry. It's not the take-out food you had last night that determines your health, but the nutrient-rich meals you eat day in, day out.

Age-friendly foods

Fresh fruit and vegetables: The most anti-aging foods you can eat are the ones that help mop up free radicals in your body (see page 16). It's no surprise that they're mostly fresh fruit and vegetables. Try fruits such as blueberries, blackberries, strawberries, raspberries, plums, oranges, red grapes, cherries, kiwi fruit, pink grapefruit, apples, tomatoes, and cantaloupe melons. Vegetable choices include steamed spinach, broccoli, beets, onion, corn, eggplant, green leafy vegetables, red bell peppers, sweet potato, Brussels sprouts, and carrots.

Locally grown organic foods: Experts advise eating these as much as possible, as they provide more vitamins and minerals than non-organic (and, of course, fewer pesticides).

Good-quality protein: Eat at least once a day. Best choices are organic chicken or fresh fish, and vegetarians can get their protein from soy-based foods plus kidney beans, chickpeas, lentils, peas, and eggs. Nuts (try almonds, cashews, Brazil nuts and hazelnuts) and seeds (such as pumpkin, sesame, sunflower, hemp, and linseeds) are also a good source of protein and provide important essential fatty acids (see over).

Raw foods: Eat more of these, which are high in nutrients and fiber. And experiment. A large proportion of our diet comes from just 19 foods, but the greater the variety of food you eat, the more nutrients you'll consume.

Water: Don't wait until you're dehydrated to down a glass of water. The mechanism that makes you thirsty becomes less effective with age, so you may have to start drinking to feel like drinking more. Make an effort to drink at least four to six large glasses of water a day (about two quarts), and your skin will feel softer by the end of it. And choose room-temperature water as ice-cold chills your stomach, making it more difficult for you to absorb nutrients.

Age-enemy foods

Sugar: This is not only very addictive, but also very aging. It wreaks havoc with your digestive system and also destroys collagen production, causing premature aging. Sugar is in most processed foods, not to mention soft drinks, chips, cakes, cookies, and chocolate, which all contain large amounts. If you feel sleepy after a meal, chances are you're suffering a sugar overload. Cut down on processed TV dinners, canned foods, and your intake of "white" foods (think bread, rice, pasta), as these are all highly processed and lacking in the goodness of their brown alternatives.

Alcohol: Alcohol extracts water from every cell in your body, causing dehydration and accelerated aging. It also generates large amounts of aging free radicals and strains your liver, causing a build-up of toxins that shows in your skin as wrinkles and broken blood vessels. One or two glasses of red wine can have a positive antioxidant benefit (young red wines are better than oak-aged), but excessive alcohol can result in many health problems, from depression to fatigue. If you like a drink, make sure you eat foods that cleanse and support the liver, including broccoli, artichokes, cauliflower, beets, radishes, and fennel. And drink dandelion-root tea, a great liver cleanser.

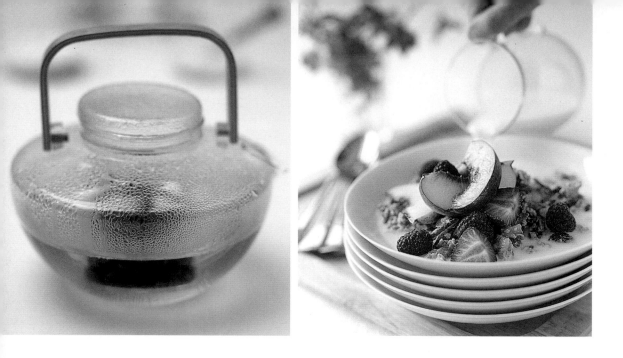

Simple Long-life Eating Habits

Really enjoy everything you eat

Most importantly, stop eating the minute you stop enjoying it. One of the simplest ways to prolong your life is to eat less, so choose smaller portions of great-tasting food and stop eating when you're full. This probably means eating slower, too, so your brain has a chance to realize you've had enough.

Make time for breakfast

In the morning your digestive juices are ready for food, so eat now or you could eventually weaken your stomach. Skipping breakfast also slows down your metabolism in order to save energy, because your body has no food to draw energy from; plus, eating all your meals later means you end up consuming calories that have nowhere useful to go.

Switch from coffee to green tea

Caffeine raises levels of cortisol (the stress hormone) and insulin, which both accelerate aging. But green tea is full of antioxidants that do wonders for the skin (see page 16) and also help speed up your metabolism, plus reduce the risk of heart disease and cancer. Green tea is an acquired taste, so look for varieties with apple, mint, or lemon, which will make the switch far sweeter.

Eat essential fats for wrinkle-free skin

Forget expensive skin creams. Essential fatty acids (EFAs) are the best investment for supple, hydrated skin with fewer wrinkles. They nourish the skin, acting as internal moisturizers to keep it soft and smooth. Symptoms of EFA deficiency actually include many common aging conditions such as dry skin, fatigue, allergies, poor memory, and inflammatory conditions (inflammation triggers most disease associated with aging, from Alzheimer's to arthritis).

There are two main types of EFAs—omegas 3 and 6. One of the best sources of omega 3 is oily fish such as mackerel, wild salmon, sardines, tuna, and herring, and seeds such as linseeds, walnuts, hemp, and pumpkin. Omega 6 is found in walnut and sesame oils and nuts like walnuts, Brazil nuts, pecans, and almonds (but not peanuts). Another option is Udo's Choice Ultimate Oil Blend, which is made from organic flax, sunflower, and sesame seeds and can be used in salad dressings or drizzled over cooked food (see Directory).

And don't mistake EFAs for the type of fat that ends up on your hips. EFAs actually encourage weight loss by increasing your metabolism to help burn stored fat, and they also help suppress appetite and decrease cravings for sweets and starchy foods (see over for more on weight loss).

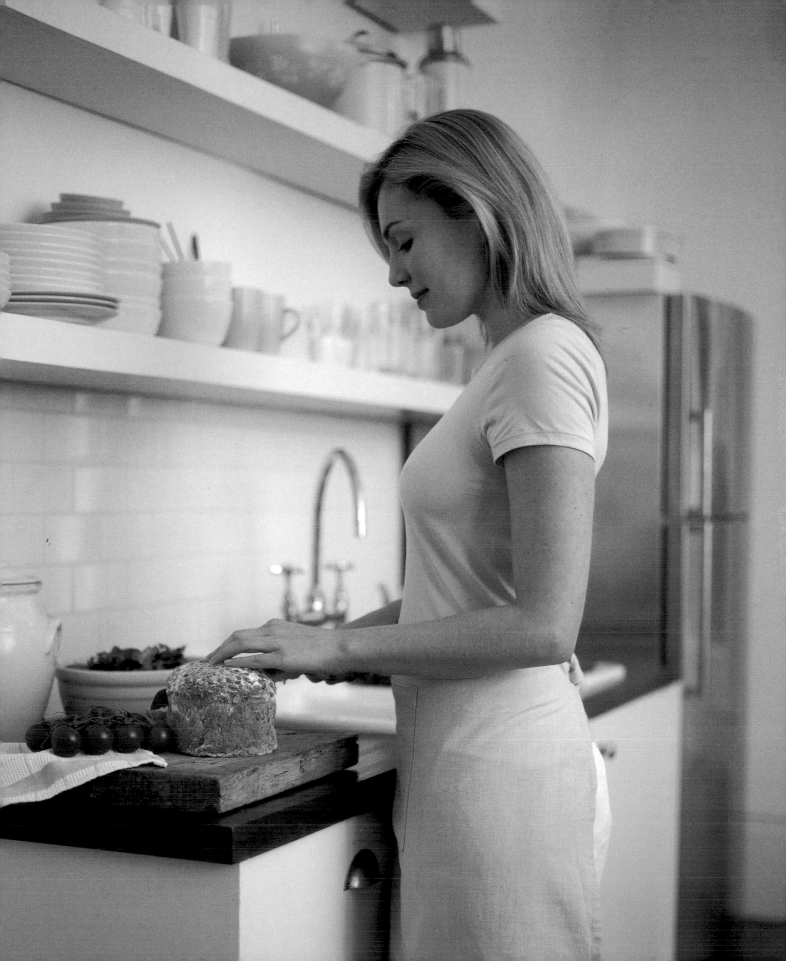

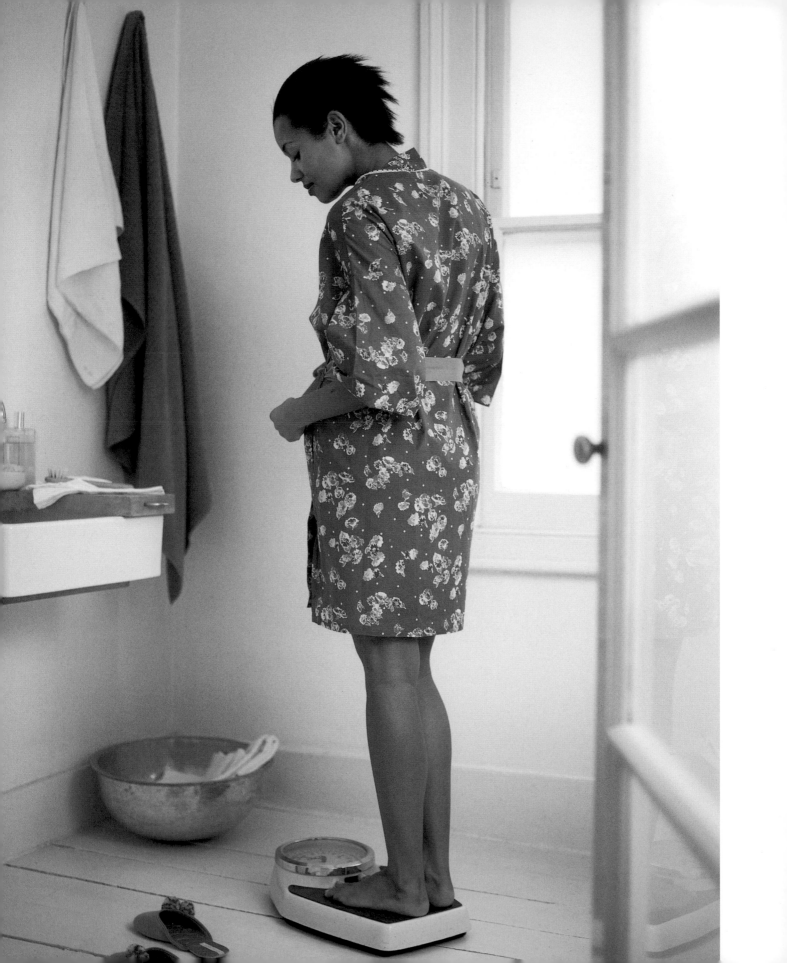

Do you Have to Put on Weight?

Being overweight significantly reduces your life expectancy, which is why you rarely see an obese person over 70. Extra weight not only puts stress on your joints, circulation, and internal organs, it can also increase your risk of serious health problems such as heart disease, arthritis, high blood pressure, diabetes, and stroke.

Many people presume that getting older means getting fatter, but middle-aged spread is not inevitable. A shift in hormones during the menopause means you may be more likely to store fat around your stomach rather than your hips, but the real reason we put on weight as we age is because most of us become less active.

This means that the majority of us can choose what we weigh at almost any age. But we can't do it with traditional weight-loss diets, or "slimming" foods that are high in sugar and sweeteners (which can actually increase your appetite and slow weight loss—see, it wasn't your lack of willpower). Around 90% of people who go on a diet put the weight back on within two years, and many go on to gain even more. Yo-yo dieting also destroys lean body mass, so when you gain the weight back, expect it to be fat, not muscle.

Instead, stop thinking diet, and start thinking healthy eating. By suddenly restricting the calories you eat, your body simply slows down your metabolism to compensate for the shortage. So forget the protein-only, blood type, and zone diets. The only thing you need to remember to maintain a healthy weight is this: good food makes you thinner.

How to maintain a healthy weight

* Eat a large variety of healthy foods you enjoy (see pages 64–65) and you'll see this as a lifelong, lifestyle choice, rather than a diet you can't wait to come off.
* Eating well will give you the energy your body needs to keep moving. Exercise is crucial for maintaining a healthy weight as it boosts metabolism and muscle mass, which in turn increases the number of calories you burn. To keep motivated, exercise needs to be enjoyable, and there really is something for everyone (see pages 92–95).

* The usual suspects are (no surprise) also the things that stop you maintaining your best weight. The roll call: refined carbohydrates (it's the white ones that cause weight gain, not the unrefined ones like whole-wheat bread and pasta); fried foods; processed foods (these disrupt blood sugar levels and are also very addictive); high-fat take-out foods (especially Indian sauce dishes); full-fat versions of milk, cheese, and butter; and desserts. Remember, it's the food you eat every day that makes the difference, not the odd hot fudge sundae you have as a treat.
* Drinking lots of water is vital to losing weight, not least because when you feel hungry it's often your body trying to tell you it needs more water. Try reaching for a glass of water instead of a snack between meals, and see if you still feel hungry afterwards.

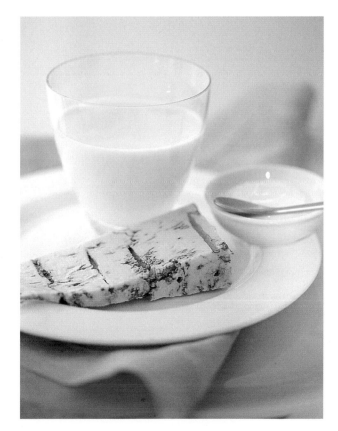

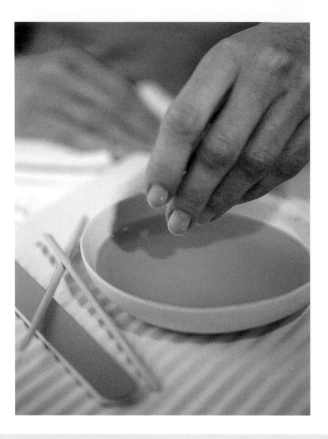
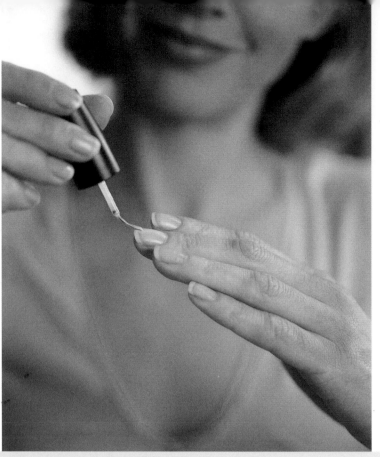

Hands of Time

It's no wonder hands and nails age fast when you add up how many times they're dunked in water, drenched with chemical cleaning products, and baked in the sun with no protection. The skin on your hands is also thinner than that on your face, so there's less fat to disguise wrinkles and veins, and less moisture to keep your skin hydrated: a recipe for accelerated aging.

Nail problems

Nails are a great barometer of health and can show up many nutritional deficiencies. Cereals, brown rice, eggs, lentils, peas, nuts, and leafy green vegetables are all important for nail health, as they're rich in B vitamins. And don't forget essential fatty acids (see page 66), which nourish nails from the inside.

What your nails are telling you

★ White spots show a lack of zinc, not calcium as is often thought. Foods high in zinc include walnuts, hazelnuts, Brazil nuts, oily fish, linseeds, and sunflower, pumpkin, and sesame seeds. White spots can also mean your intake of sugar, alcohol, and/or junk food is too high.

★ Brittle, splitting nails are a sign of silica deficiency (silica is found in all high-fiber foods, vegetables, and wholegrains).

★ Soft, peeling nails signal calcium deficiency. Up your calcium intake by eating cheese, milk, yogurt, broccoli, and spinach.

★ Longitudinal ridges can be a sign of low stomach acid. Try drinking a glass of warm water with two teaspoons of apple cider vinegar and a squeeze of lemon every morning.

★ Horizontal ridges on your nails are due to a lack of calcium (see above) and/or magnesium (find it in milk, yogurt, artichokes, and whole-wheat bread). They can also denote a too-high stress level.

Replace lost moisture by **soaking** your nails in oil (try **jojoba**, olive, or almond oil) once a week.

How to stop your hands giving your age away

Queen of nails, Jessica Vartoughian (see Directory), whose clients include Julia Roberts, Madonna, Demi Moore, and Jodie Foster, has this advice for beautiful hands and nails after a certain age.

* Shorter, well-groomed nails are far more flattering on older hands than long talons. The best shape is a round oval, which follows the shape of your half-moon.
* Nails get thicker and harder as you age, so it's unlikely you'll need a strengthening product. Instead, aim to replace lost moisture by soaking your nails in oil (try jojoba, olive, or almond oil) once or twice a week. Warm the oil in a saucer placed over a pan of boiling water, and then pour it into a cup before soaking for 10 minutes.
* To double the effect, soak your nails last thing at night, then massage the oil into your hands, put on a pair of cotton gloves, and go to bed. You'll be amazed how soft your skin feels in the morning.
* A quick and easy way to give your hands the heat experience is to keep your hand cream by a radiator.
* Use a hand cream with an SPF15 to protect your hands from age spots caused by UV exposure. You may even find existing sun spots begin to fade, as some sun damage can be reversed once skin is no longer exposed.
* To remove yellow stains from nails (these are caused by wearing colored polish with no base coat, and smoking), soak them in a cup of warm water and the juice of one lemon for 15 minutes.
* Wear rubber gloves when doing the dishes or house-cleaning, gardening gloves when doing outside work, and warm gloves once the temperature drops, to protect hands from the dehydrating cold and wind.
* Rather than buffing, which removes layers of nail, massage a cuticle oil or cream into your nails and cuticles daily. This will do the same job of increasing circulation and growth.

* Multi-task by applying cream, putting on a pair of disposable gloves, and then putting rubber gloves over the top. The heat generated while you do the dishes will encourage the moisture to sink in and leave your hands super-soft.
* If protruding veins are a problem, hold up your hands and shake, bring them down and repeat three times. This will release the veins—it's a favorite with celebrities before they step out onto the red carpet.
* As we get older, women often choose nude or brown-based shades of polish, but these aren't good on older skins. Far more flattering are strong sheers or a full-blown bright shade.

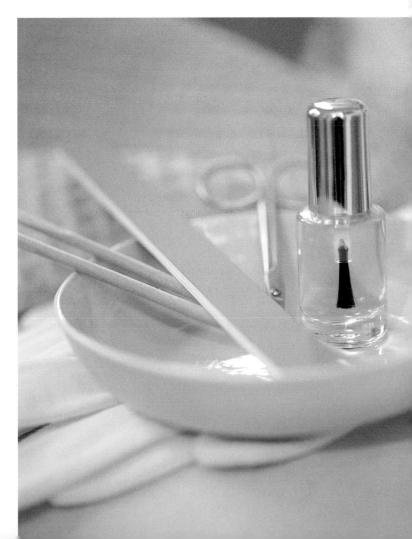

How to Keep your Feet Fit (and Fabulous)

The average person walks approximately 115,000 miles in a lifetime (that's more than four times the circumference of the globe), and your poor feet live in shoes for 16 hours a day (which is two thirds of a lifetime). No surprise, then, that millions of us seek medical advice for our feet each year and, thanks to a love of forbidding footwear, women's feet get run down quicker than men's and suffer far more problems.

Fit foot advice

* The skin on your feet is already the least lubricated on your body, and it only gets drier with age. For a deep moisture treat, place a pair of cotton socks on the radiator. Before going to bed, massage a teaspoon of olive oil into your skin and slip the warm socks on so the oil penetrates deeply as you sleep.

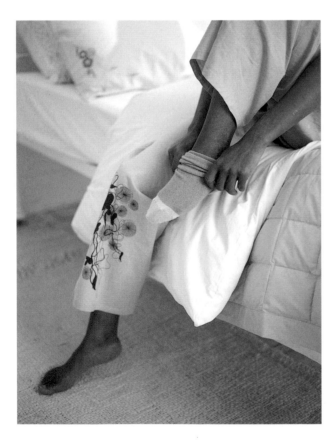

* High heels put added pressure on the balls of your feet, toes, and joints. Some catwalk models resort to Restylane injections in the balls of their feet to give them extra padding and prevent that burning sensation. A far more sensible option is to use padded inserts (available from drug stores), which cushion the ball of your foot and prevent it from slipping forward in your shoe.
* Minimize the risk of heel-induced injuries by doing squats and calf rises to strengthen your leg muscles. Exercising your feet will also increase joint mobility and strength. Sit with feet outstretched and rotate your ankles in a circle in either direction 10 times. Then curl up your toes and stretch them out 10 times on each foot, or have fun trying to pick up a pencil off the floor.
* Drain away the excess fluid that causes swollen ankles and feet by propping your legs against the wall at a 45-degree angle for 10 minutes.

Smart shoe shopping

* Wearing the right size shoes improves your posture and helps prevent back problems later in life—your toes should be able to wiggle in the shoe. Also, vary heel height daily to keep the muscles in your feet and calves flexible.
* Walking in new shoes causes the majority of blisters, so always break shoes in by wearing them around the house for a short time. Avoid mass-produced shoes made of cheap material, as they have trouble adapting to the shape of your feet, making them more likely to rub, causing blisters and pain.
* Feet can suffer the equivalent of middle-aged spread, flattening down to become up to a whole size bigger. They can also change size due to weight gain or loss, hard work, and pregnancy, so it's worth getting your feet measured once a year after the age of 40.
* Around 90% of us have feet of different sizes (which is another reason for a regular measure). Always buy shoes to fit the larger foot and use a padded inner sole to make the other one fit snugly.

Around 90% of us have feet of **different** sizes. Always buy shoes to fit the **larger** foot.

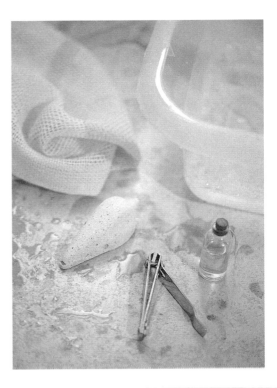

Pamper your feet with this simple pedicure

1 Soak your feet in warm water for five minutes.

2 Cut toenails straight across and then file down any sharp edges (clipping the corners to give a round shape can lead to ingrown toenails).

3 Push back cuticles while they're soft with an orange stick.

4 Remove hard skin from around the heels and balls of your feet with a foot file. Do this when your feet are dry or you could remove too much skin.

5 Massage in a moisturizer and blot away any excess.

6 "Squeak" the nails with a washcloth dunked in cold water in preparation for painting. Twist a strip of kitchen towel and weave it through your toes to separate them.

7 Apply a base coat and then two coats of color (the more strokes you use to apply your polish, the longer-lasting the result). Reapply your top coat every two days for a pedicure that should last for up to two months.

How to Keep Hold of your Teeth

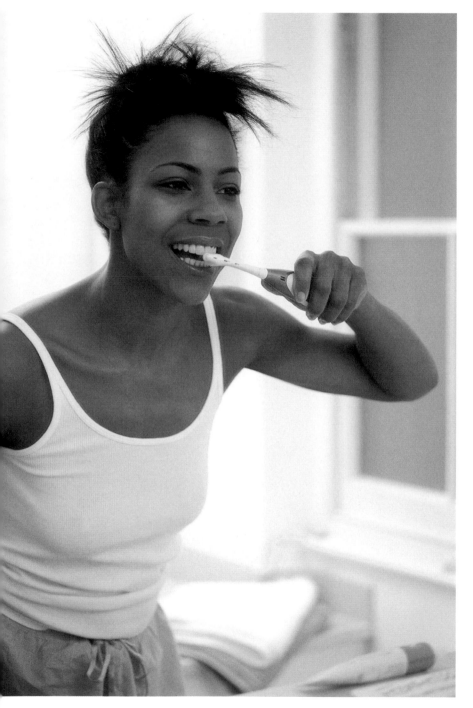

Age isn't kind to your teeth, which is why good oral hygiene is even more important now. The older you get, the duller your teeth become, due to years of red wine, coffee, and herbal tea drinking (if you notice your cups are stained after certain drinks, the same is happening to your teeth). Your gums also shrink, giving you that long-in-the-tooth look, and teeth can get worn down after years of night-time grinding. In addition to this list of woes, your gums are also more prone to disease as you age, which can lead to bad breath and worse. With one in seven people losing all their teeth before they're 50, you need to know how to stop the rot.

Everyday dental essentials

* Brush your teeth twice a day to prevent the build-up of plaque on the surface. It's much better to spend longer brushing gently with a soft-bristled brush than brushing hard and fast, which can cause erosion. For best results, use an electric toothbrush (any electric action is better than your manual technique), and replace bristles once they're splayed.

* Floss every night to remove food from the places your toothbrush can't reach. And don't go easy if your gums bleed, as this is the first stage of gum disease. If you continue to floss, you'll remove the plaque and stop the rot. Regular flossing can also help you live longer, as gum disease is now linked to heart disease (bacteria from the mouth can be absorbed into the bloodstream, ending up in the heart valves).

* You probably think brushing after a meal is the best option, but it's actually better to brush before eating, as food acids soften

enamel, making it easy for you to remove a layer. And the less enamel there is, the yellower your teeth become, as the underlying dentine shows through. If you want to freshen your mouth right after eating, rinse with water, which will also help neutralize the acids.

★ Ironically, most "whitening" toothpastes contain abrasives that work by scratching the surface of the teeth, causing eventual erosion (and therefore yellowing).

★ Fluoride is actually a by-product of the fertilizer industry and known to be carcinogenic. Far better are natural toothpastes (see Directory), which are not only less abrasive but also free of fluoride, artificial sweeteners, preservatives, colorings, and other synthetic additives. Unsurprisingly, they taste nicer, too.

★ Beware sugary food and drinks. They weaken enamel, allowing bacteria to enter the teeth and cause decay. And cut down on soft drinks (including sparkling water), which can also erode enamel.

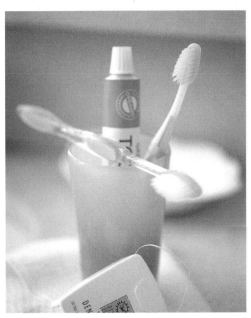

Brightening your smile

★ For a quick fix, visit the hygienist at your dentist for a 30-minute scale and polish. While not exactly pleasurable, you really do leave with a brighter smile, thanks to a good brush with an abrasive paste that removes stains and restores whiteness.

★ Do-it-yourself teeth-bleaching kits are now widely available, but don't expect dramatic results as the strength of the bleaching solution is not as strong as the one your dentist can sell you (dentists use hydrogen peroxide, while most home kits use softer-acting sodium chloride). The solution is squeezed into a tray that fits over your teeth, but this is a standard size rather than being custom-made, as it would be at your dentist (see over).

★ You can make your teeth look whiter by wearing lipstick shades that contrast with yellow. That means avoiding anything with a yellow or orange undertone, such as coral and some browns, and going for colors with a cool tone, such as shades of berry and burgundy, plus blue-based reds and pinks.

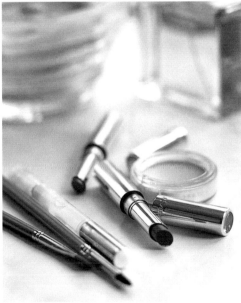

Natural toothpastes are free of fluoride, artificial sweeteners, and colorings. They taste nicer, too.

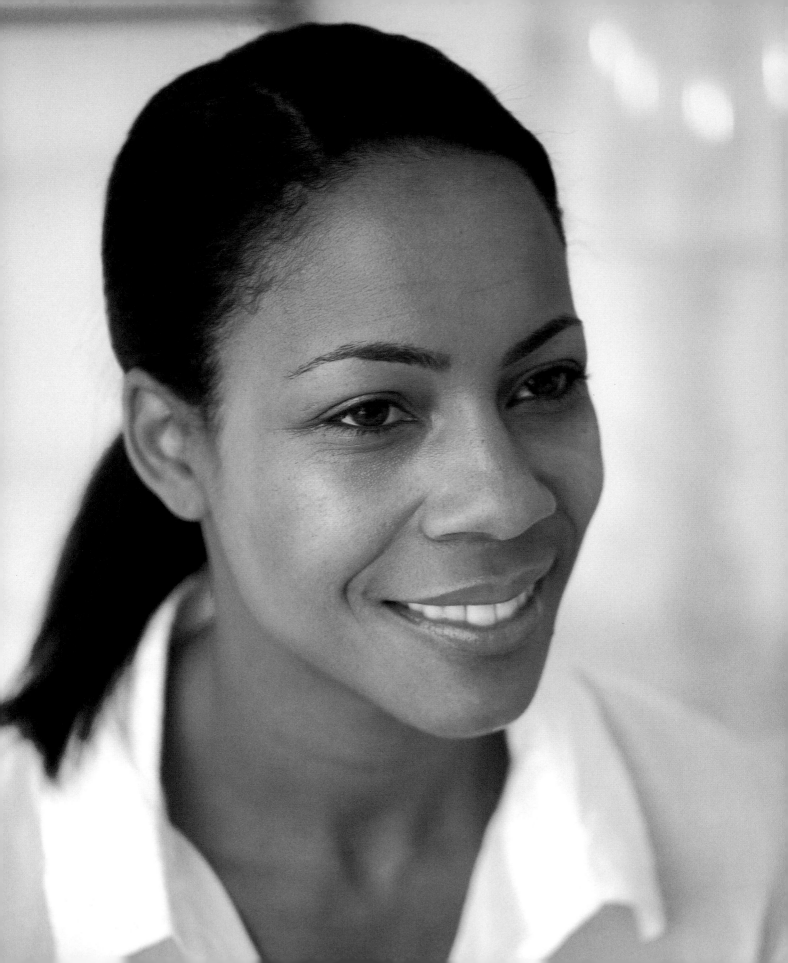

How a Dentist can Make you Look Younger

If you put your hand over your mouth when you smile or clamp your lips together in photos, then you're the perfect candidate for cosmetic dentistry. The following treatments can work like a mini facelift, with people saying how good you look but not quite knowing why. Unfortunately, cosmetic dentistry comes at a high price, and it's important to find a good dentist to ensure the work doesn't cause problems later. It's not taught at dental school, which means dentists must train further after graduation, making it extra important that you do your research.

Ensure your dentist is an Accredited Member of the American Academy of Cosmetic Dentistry (see Directory), which will mean that they have completed extensive post-graduate training in cosmetic dentistry. Always visit your chosen dentist for a consultation first. Many offer computer imagery so you can see a picture of yourself with your new smile before going ahead.

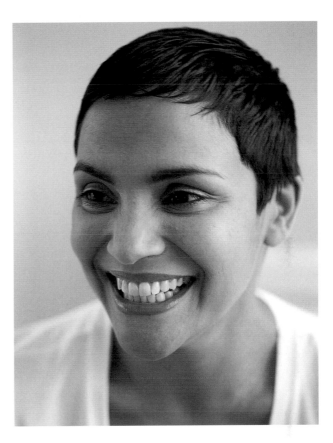

Teeth whitening

The most popular method uses a tray and can be done yourself at home. Your dentist takes an impression of your teeth and a custom-built tray is made. At home, you squeeze in a tiny drop of hydrogen peroxide gel for each tooth and wear it for up to an hour or overnight for one to two weeks (depending upon instructions). Expect to pay in the region of $500, with top-up kits also available.

The second technique is light or laser-power whitening. Your gums and lips are coated with silicone for protection and then a concentrated solution is applied to your teeth. A high-intensity light is shone on them for an hour, which penetrates the enamel and draws out stains. The procedure is not exactly painful, but if you have a high level of sensitivity, you could take a painkiller beforehand. Laser whitening is more expensive than the tray method above (but only takes an hour). Both these methods can improve the brightness of your teeth by up to 70%, with results lasting up to three years. Six-monthly hygienist appointments will prolong the results by removing stains and giving teeth a polish.

Veneers and crowns

A godsend for crooked or badly discolored teeth, they also bulk out teeth to provide a plumping, anti-aging effect on your face. Veneers are tailor-made porcelain covers that are fitted over teeth and last up to 15 years. The front of the tooth is first filed down and the veneer is glued over the top. Don't underestimate how different these can make you look, but the price is high (starting at around $1,300 for two). Crowns are the traditional way of repairing problem teeth, and are needed if teeth are more seriously misshapen. The tooth is ground down to a peg and a replica fitted over the top. More modern methods mean crowns no longer have that telltale shadow around the gum and will last longer, too (up to 20 years). Crowns cost about $800 per tooth.

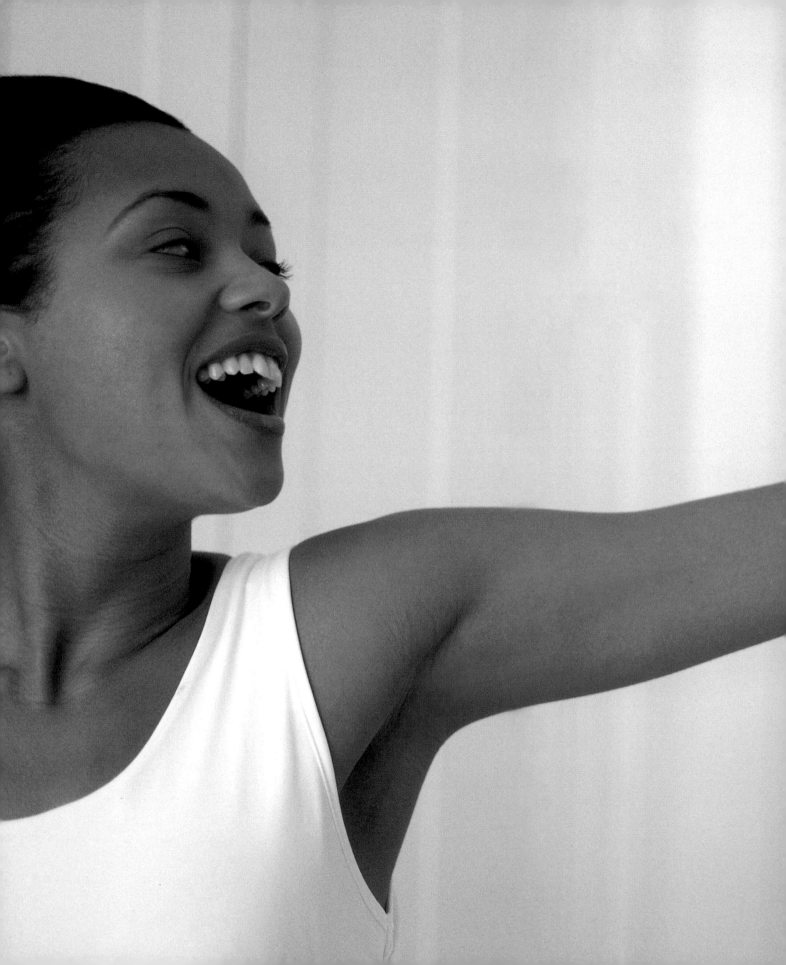

Ageless Energy
Keeping yourself fabulously fit

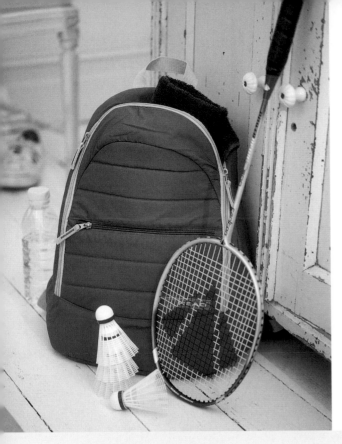

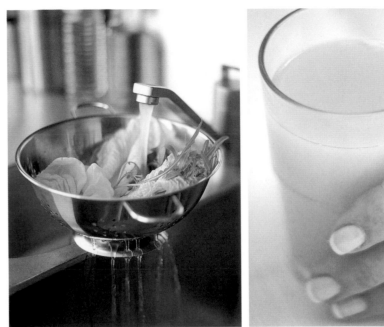

High-energy Habits

One in ten of us complains of constant tiredness, but feeling exhausted isn't just inconvenient—it's your body's way of telling you to do something about it before you get sick. Persistent tiredness can cause everything from depression and anemia to chronic fatigue syndrome, plus if you feel drained all the time you're going to look it, too! It's easy to blame lack of energy on age, but your energy levels actually don't need to drop as you get older. How lively you feel is more in your control than you think.

Eat for energy

We need a constant top-up of quality nutrients so our bodies can convert them to fuel, and making changes to your diet can have a massive effect on your energy levels. The simplest way to increase your stamina is to eat a healthy breakfast. Protein helps wake up your brain, making eggs the perfect way to start the day. Dehydration is a major cause of fatigue, so make sure you drink the recommended eight glasses of water a day. For sustained energy, you can't beat protein-rich foods like lean meat, cheese, oily fish, and tofu (vegetarians can choose brown rice, oats, lentils, nuts, and seeds). And eat more fresh fruit and vegetables, or whizz them up in a blender to make energy-packed drinks. For a sustained midday energy boost, go for dried fruit like dates, apricots, and raisins, or pumpkin and sunflower seeds. And snack on potassium-packed foods such as oranges, bananas, and peanut butter.

Eat for endurance

Any food that gives you a quick-fix energy boost will soon send you crashing. Sugar, caffeine, sodas (including so-called energy drinks), and white foods like bread, pasta, and cakes will drain your energy. Save wheat-based meals for evenings, as they may make you sleepy. Smaller meals eaten throughout the day will keep your energy levels constant, unlike a large meal, which will wear you out digesting it.

Allow yourself **one day** to do as little as humanly possible. Relax in your pyjamas. Go for a **walk**. **Read** in bed. Have a long bath. Indulge yourself.

Keep fit

Never underestimate the power of exercising, which will up your energy levels for at least two hours afterwards (see pages 88–95). Just a 30-minute walk in the fresh air will produce enough oxygen to boost your energy levels. Sufficient sleep is also vital for energy (see pages 96–99).

Detox your diet

Reduce the number of toxins in your body, because they produce energy-sapping free radicals (see pages 62–63).

Recharge your batteries

Low energy can also be a sign of what's going on inside your head. The red blood cells of depressed and stressed people carry less oxygen, and the less oxygen in your blood, the less energy in your body. Stop asking too much of yourself (see page 86) and take regular time off. You only have a certain amount of energy, so if you keep giving out, then you're going to need to recharge. Allow yourself one day to do as little as humanly possible. Relax in your pyjamas. Go for a walk. Read in bed. Have a long bath. Indulge yourself and *be* rather than *do* for one day.

Nurture feel-good friendships

We connect with each other through energy (see over), so don't hang around with negative people who drain you, and save time for friends who make you feel good. If you have to spend time with someone who saps your energy, imagine putting up an invisible barrier to keep their negativity away.

Expend energy wisely

Managing your energy is far more important than managing your time, so use it consciously. Every day, decide how you're going to use your reserve. Ask yourself: Is what I'm doing important to me right now? Look at your life and see what you really value in it, then prioritize those people and activities (see pages 118–119 for more time-savvy advice).

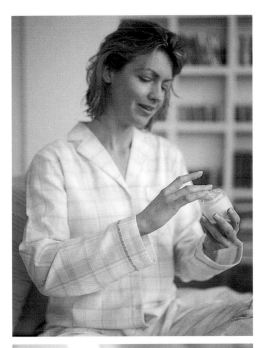

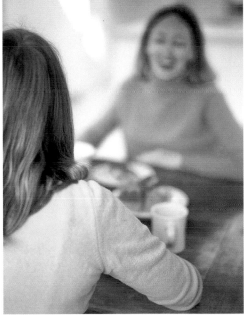

Turn up your Frequency

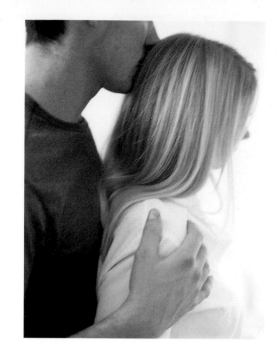

When you meet someone for the first time, it's their energy you're attracted to—or not. If you're introduced to a new person who does nothing but moan, chances are you'll be desperate to get away. The energy that flows out of us comes from our emotions, and like attracts like. If we spend our time feeling "up," our emotions send out high-frequency vibrations that draw anything (or anyone) with the same frequency right back to us. But if we spend our time thinking about what's wrong, those low-frequency feelings are going to attract more of the same. Just as tuning forks in the same room set off others with a matching vibration, so you attract more of your own.

It takes only seconds to link up energetically to whatever you're focusing on, which makes our thoughts incredibly powerful. Luckily you can manipulate them when they're not making you feel so good, and every time you alter your thoughts in a positive way, you're raising your energy level. Be aware of how a thought is making you feel: good or bad? Then ask yourself: If it was up to me, how would I choose to feel about this situation? Choose something better and you become the creator of your thoughts rather than the victim.

So, how do you stop a negative thought? Simply by thinking about something that gives you pleasure. Our bodies contain endorphins, which manufacture positive emotions, and the spontaneous release you get when you're happy can be manipulated just by thinking a happy thought. The moment you catch yourself focusing on what is wrong, *make* yourself find something good to think about (this can be anything that gives you a good feeling) and stay there until you feel your mood begin to change. Then make this thought more vivid in your mind until you begin to feel exactly what you experienced at the time.

The only power that problems have over us is the power we give them. If you want something, it's no good staying stuck in what you haven't got. You've got to feel the excitement of what you want. So, if you're desperate for a new job, don't obsess about how much you hate your current one, but get excited at the prospect of a better one. And if your partner is distant, don't focus on what he doesn't do for you, but on what he does—and what you'd like him to do in the future. Both of these are far more likely to get you what you want. Prospective employers will respond to you more positively (not to mention your current employer). And your partner will want to spend time with the positive you, rather than the moaning version. The only way to stop the not-so-good stuff in your life getting worse is to stop focusing on it. After all, do you want to be that party guest everyone tries to escape, or the person everyone wants to know?

It takes **seconds** to link up energetically to what you're focusing on, which makes our **thoughts** incredibly powerful. Every time you alter your thoughts in a **positive** way, you raise your energy.

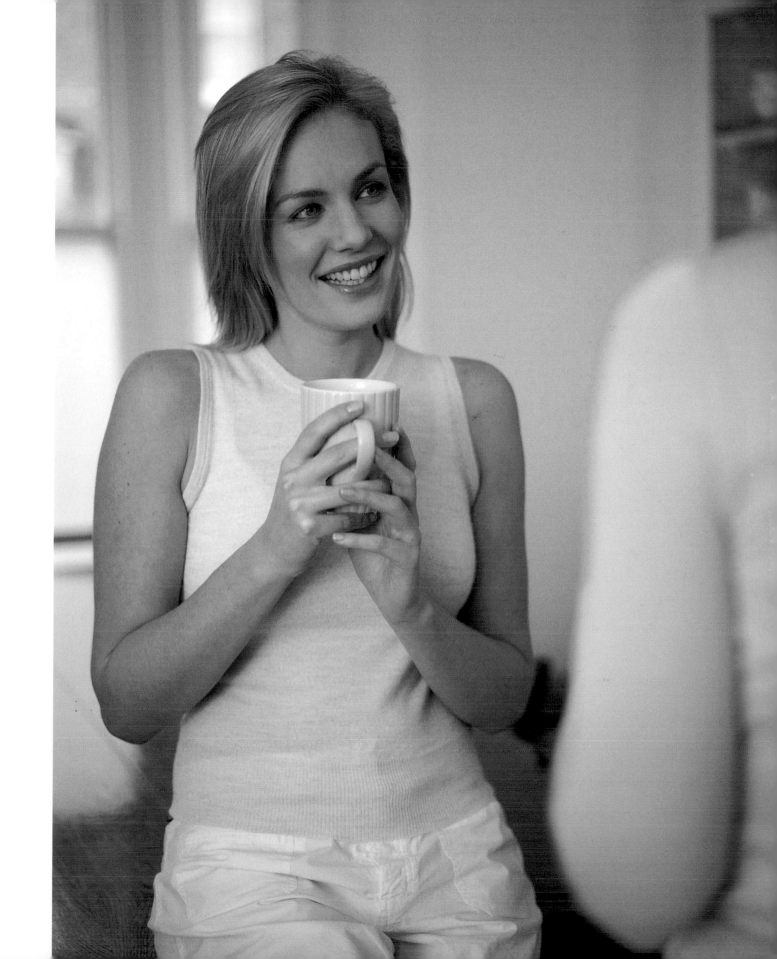

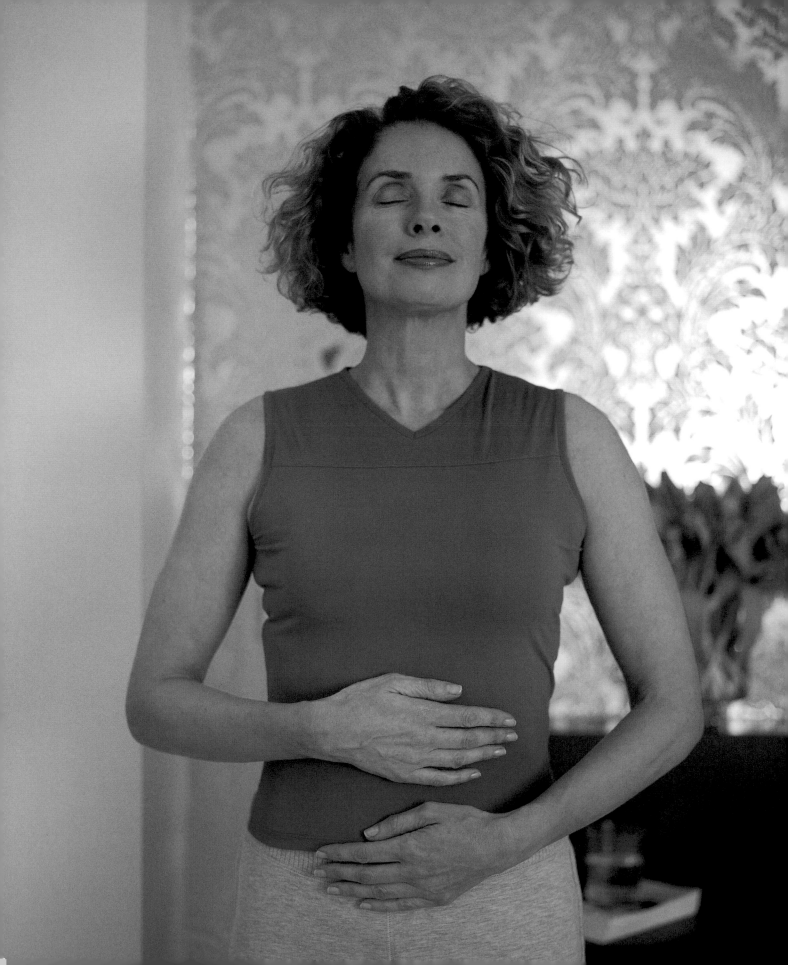

Take a Deep Breath

Anti-aging breathing

Every time you breathe, you inhale oxygen into your bloodstream and exhale toxic waste from your cells. Oxygen has a healthy, alkaline effect, which energizes your whole body, improves skin tone, and fights disease, while carbon dioxide is acid-forming. This sounds perfect, but daily stress causes most of us to take in only a third of our lung capacity, which means a lot of waste is never expelled. Shallow breathing can cause your lungs to lose their elasticity, leading to problems such as bronchitis and asthma. But begin breathing properly and you'll instantly look and feel better. Abdominal breathing works as a free anti-ager, by not only energizing your whole body but also expanding your left-out lower lungs. It also encourages better digestion and helps fight the bacterial and fungal infections that thrive when there's not much oxygen around. Wherever you are, try this belly breath now.

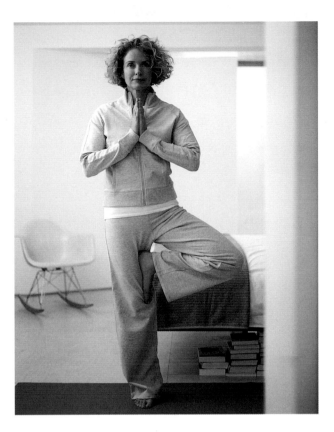

1 Put your hand just below your tummy button, breathe in through your nose and feel your stomach inflate.
2 Breathe lightly and gently so your shoulders stay relaxed, then exhale through your mouth, feeling your hand fall.

Do this any time you're stressed and you'll notice how much more relaxed you feel. It's also the perfect way to end the day, especially when you're lying in bed at night, as it calms your heart rate, helping you drift off to sleep.

Long term, improve your breathing with yoga, Pilates, or a gentle martial art; they are all based on movement with slow, steady breathing. Or sing along to a CD, which will increase your lung capacity and make you breathe more deeply.

Stay-young meditation

Regular meditation reduces the amount of adrenaline and cortisol, the stress hormones that speed up aging, in your body. It also increases the level of DHEA, a hormone that declines with age (low levels are linked to a risk of heart disease, osteoporosis, and breast cancer). In studies, a group of 50-year-old meditators even experienced a 12-year decrease in their biological age (see pages 8–9). Meditation also calms your mind and eases muscle tension, making it the perfect slow-down in a speedy world.

The basis of all meditation is switching your brainwaves from their normal busy beta state to a more relaxed alpha state. Just like abdominal breathing, meditation is free, but how do you find the time? Simple. Rather than waiting for that uninterrupted, quiet moment in life (which never comes), use meditation to switch off from an otherwise mad world. It's the perfect way to spend your commute or any other "dead time." Just sit comfortably with arms and legs uncrossed and eyes closed. Start to breathe gently and imagine your body relaxing. Transcendental meditation gives you a mantra to repeat silently over and over to help quiet your internal chatter (any two-syllable, soothing word will do). As you repeat it, focus on your breathing, which will slow and settle in time with your words. When thoughts (or external noises) break through, simply acknowledge them and go back to your mantra. Aim for 15–20 minutes, and come out of it slowly, as your mind will want a few minutes to readjust. This is also a great technique to try when you're lying in bed with a racing brain that won't let you sleep.

Energy Sappers

If you are one of the types below, your behavior will be seriously sapping your energy, so do yourself a favor and stop sabotaging yourself. It may take time to change your (lifelong?) habit, but the results will change your life forever.

Perfectionist

You're making your life far harder than it has to be by constantly aiming for the impossible. You know you can't really be perfect, and by fearing achieving anything less, you probably never start (or finish) half of what you'd like to. Think of someone you admire. Are they perfect? Probably not, but you still respect them, so why shouldn't others feel the same about you? You need to think about how much your perfectionism affects your life and whether it makes you happy. Again, it probably doesn't. So here's what to do. Instead of aiming for perfection, just aim to do your best. There may be minor imperfections, but are the consequences really that terrible? Rather than using your perfectionism to procrastinate ("I'll just do it one more time"), just decide to learn from your mistakes so you don't repeat them next time.

Control freak

Control freaks are very hard to live with. Your message to others is that you can't trust them to do anything as well as you can. A need for control often hides a fear of feeling out of control, and the anxiety which that causes can be exhausting. How much more energy do you have to utilize, compared with others? Your first step is to understand why you seek to control your environment. All of us want to feel some measure of control over our lives, but when everything (and everyone) has to go your way, you're heading for trouble. Ask yourself: When did you feel helpless? Are you the same person now? Why do you still need to control everything to feel safe? What's the worst that can happen if you let go? Practice consciously handing over the responsibility occasionally and see what happens. Does the sky fall in, or do you just get to relax once in a while?

Adrenaline junkie

Running on adrenaline makes you speak fast and act stupid. You have no patience with others and often leave everything until the last minute. You're nearly always late and have at least four irate incidents by the time you get there. Adrenaline addicts can find they miss the stress when there's no pressure to perform, but in the long term they're heading for disaster (if not an early grave). There are never enough hours in the day, but how much time this week have you spent on activities that have no meaning to you? Aren't you more important? Often a chaotic mind is also a way to distract yourself from doing what you really want to, or facing up to a long-forgotten truth. Ask yourself: What would you regret not doing if you continue living the way you do now? Then clear some space to get started. Convincing yourself that every second of your life has to be filled is also a way to feel successful or popular. But who taught you to feel guilty for doing nothing? A much healthier plan is to decide what activities are most important to you and drop the rest, so you have time to recharge your batteries.

> Here's what to do. Instead of aiming for perfection, just aim to do your best. Rather than using your perfectionism to procrastinate, decide to learn from your mistakes so you don't repeat them.

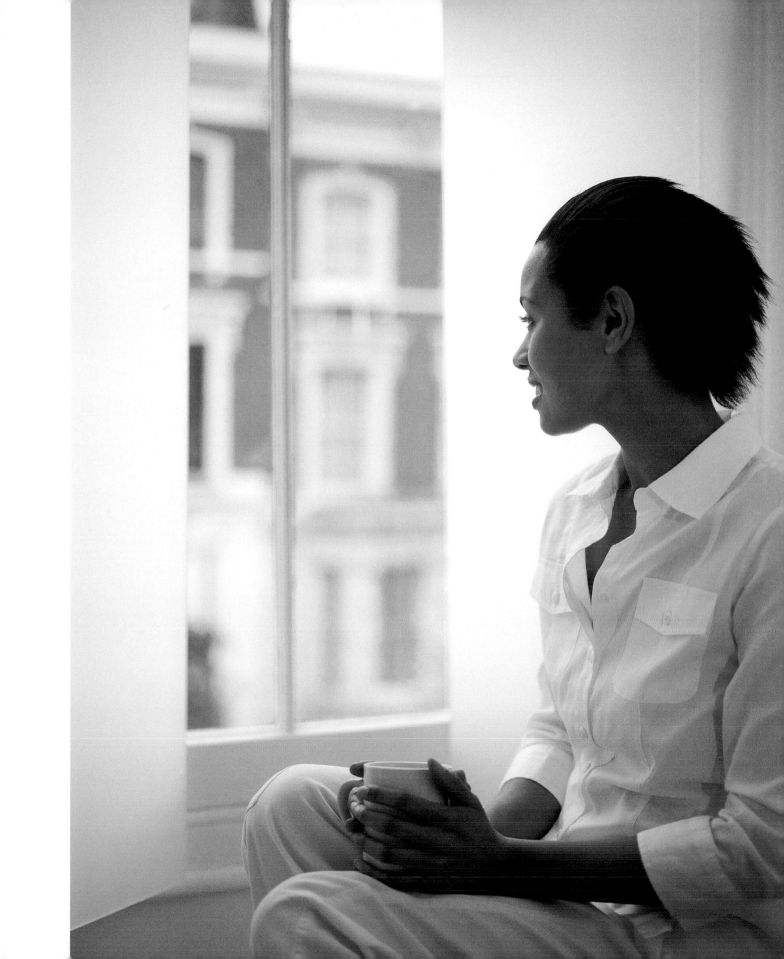

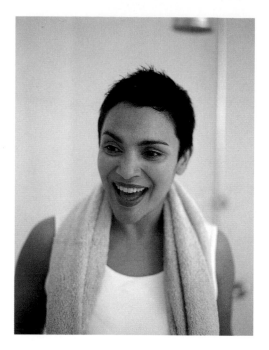

Great Reasons to Exercise

We all know what regular exercise does for the waistline, but prepare to be amazed at just how much it benefits the rest of you, including significantly slowing down the aging process. You may not want to be running marathons at 70 (although plenty of people do), but increasing your activity will help you enjoy your life more—for a whole lot longer.

1 Regular exercise increases your body's production of SOD, an anti-aging enzyme that fights the free radicals which cause cell breakdown and skin damage.

2 Exercise also raises levels of the anti-aging hormone DHEA, which has been found to help prevent everything from brain aging to heart disease, while at the same time improving your mood and energy levels.

3 The reason you feel good after exercise is because it raises levels of endorphins, the chemicals we make naturally when we're happy. These not only act as natural painkillers but also reduce tension, anxiety, and even appetite.

4 Exercise raises levels of the feel-good hormone serotonin, which helps you feel more positive. Serotonin is so effective at fighting depression that both Prozac and St. John's wort work by preventing its breakdown.

5 Even moderate exercise will strengthen your immune system, making you far less likely to catch a cold. And fitter people also recover from illnesses more quickly, whether it be a niggling sore throat or major surgery.

6 Sleep is nature's best beauty treatment (see pages 96–97). Exercisers sleep more soundly (spending extra time in the most restorative phases), and wake less often through the night, than sedentary people.

7 Active women are less likely to experience hot flushes during the menopause, and the mood-boost that exercise provides helps ease other menopausal symptoms, too.

8 Flexibility is the first thing to go with age, but gentle stretching exercises such as yoga and Pilates will keep you supple for life. As little as five minutes' stretching a day will help keep your muscles loose and limber for longer.

9 Exercise boosts your lymphatic system, which is responsible for removing toxins, and also moves important anti-aging vitamins around your body.

10 Women start losing bone mass between the ages of 30 and 40, but weight-bearing exercise such as walking keeps your bones stronger by thickening joint cartilage. Exercise also drastically reduces your risk of osteoporosis.

11 Exercise strengthens your ligaments and tendons, making couch potatoes far more likely to suffer from back and joint problems than active people who work their muscles regularly.

12 Forget not having enough energy to exercise. Raise your activity rate and you'll have more energy, not less. Anything that raises your heartbeat and gets you breathing a little faster will improve your stamina for everything else in life.

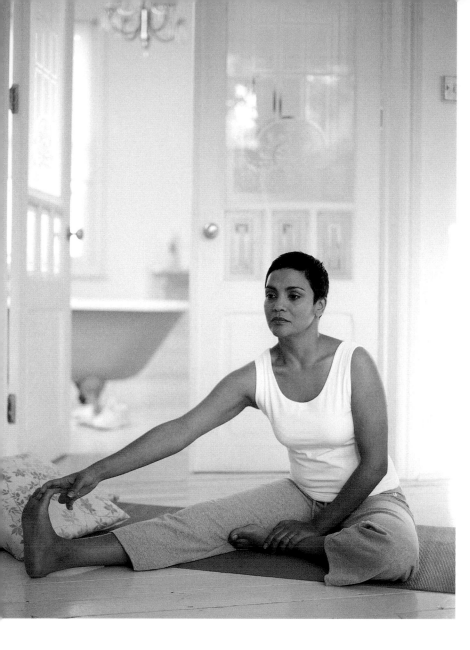

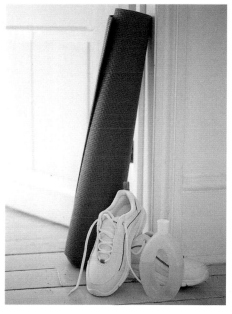

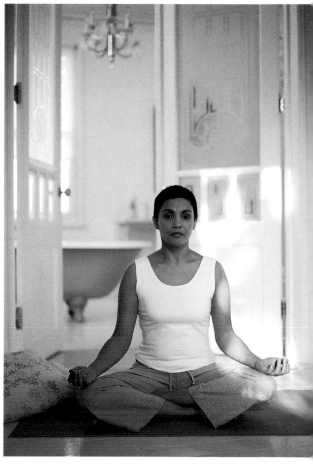

13 After 30, your metabolic rate drops by almost 5% a decade, but exercise increases it, making you burn stored fat faster even when you're relaxing.

14 Regular exercise makes your body look younger by improving your posture. When your stomach and back muscles are strong, you'll walk tall and proud instead of hunching over like an old person.

15 Exercise makes your body feel years younger. Women who exercise regularly have the strength, bone density, metabolism, flexibility, muscle bulk, and blood pressure of women 15 to 20 years younger.

How Much Exercise is Enough?

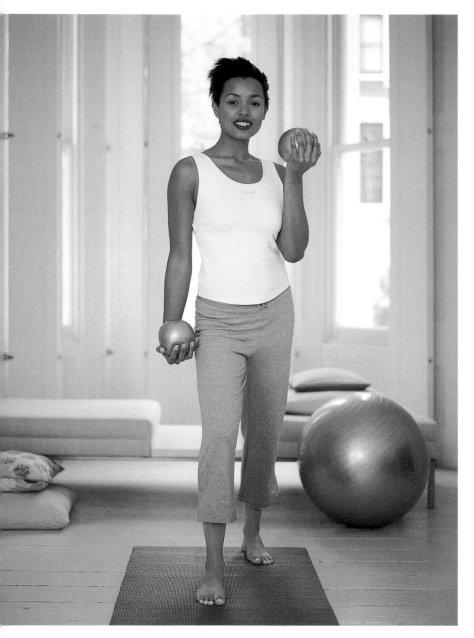

Losing muscle mass and strength is the cause of most physical signs of aging, so it's easy to see why exercise that rebuilds and strengthens muscle will instantly make you look younger. In fact, just one year of light weight training can fast-track your muscle bulk and strength, metabolism, flexibility, and certain hormone levels back by an amazing 15 to 20 years.

So how much is enough? Any exercise is better than none, so never use lack of time as an excuse not to reap the benefits. Even walking to the station every morning will increase bone density and metabolism (which is why many people put on weight after they've bought a car). Start with five minutes' brisk walking a day and you'll look and feel better almost immediately. For optimum results, exercise for 30 minutes, three to four times a week (you can drop this to twice a week once you have achieved your desired result).

Maintaining your fitness

Don't let 48 hours pass without some kind of activity, as you want to keep your metabolic rate buzzing to burn fat effectively. Exercising in the afternoon is the best time for weight loss, as your hormone levels are high, and activity at this time will help you sleep at the end of the day, too. Fitness experts also advise interval training, which simply means working harder for a few minutes, then slowing down a little before speeding up again, as this burns more calories.

Start with **five minutes'** brisk walking a day and you'll look and feel better almost **immediately**.

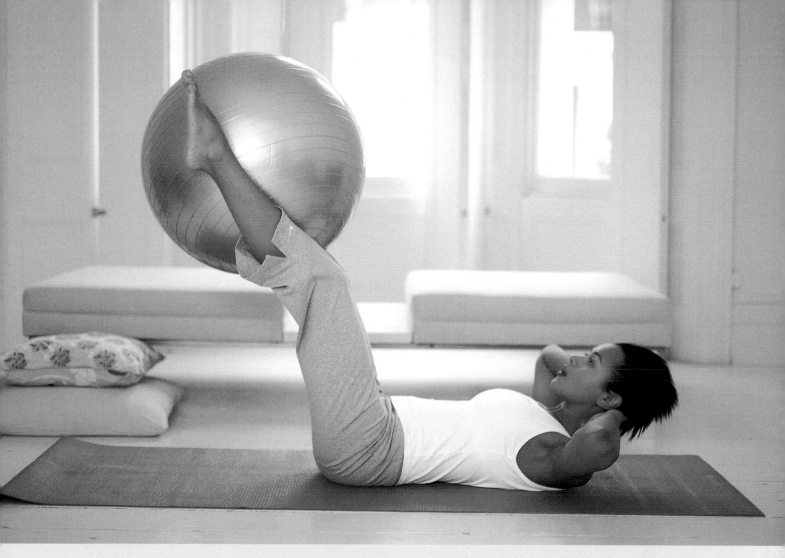

What exercise does to your hormones

Certain hormone levels decline with age, but by increasing and rebalancing them with exercise, you can literally help reverse the aging process.

* Endorphins are the most well-known hormones released as our bodies' biochemistry changes during a bout of exercise. They not only give you that feel-good factor (they are natural opiates) but also reduce anxiety and appetite. Endorphins are increased by a whopping 500% after 30 minutes of moderate aerobic exercise.

* Growth hormones decline with age and can be the cause of weight gain, low energy, dry and sagging skin, disrupted sleep, and poor concentration. Both aerobic exercise and weight training will increase your growth hormone levels after 30 minutes.

* The male hormone testosterone is important for maintaining muscle tone and strength, plus it increases your metabolic rate, helping to reduce body fat. Testosterone increases in your blood after 20 minutes of exercise and peaks after 30, staying high for up to three hours afterwards.

* The female hormone estrogen declines at the menopause and is responsible for boosting metabolism and fat breakdown. It also increases after exercise and stays high for up to four hours afterwards.

* Thyroxin speeds skin-cell renewal and boosts energy levels, helping you burn calories faster. It increases in the blood during exercise and stays high for up to three hours afterwards.

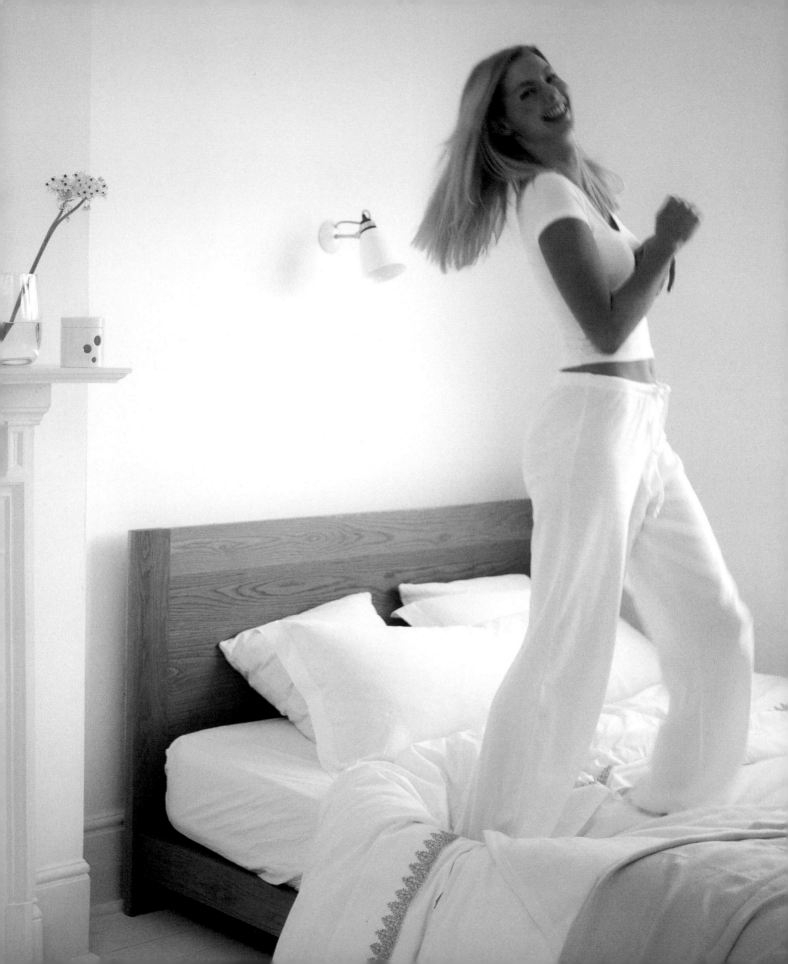

Enjoyable, Easy Exercise

Gym-based exercise can not only be incredibly boring but also very inconvenient. Not so the following, which are free, easy, simple to fit into your life—and maybe even enjoyable?

The wonder of walking

It's estimated that every minute of walking extends your life by up to two minutes. Not a bad return. In fact, walking at a brisk pace is nature's greatest fitness booster. It doesn't jar your joints like jogging, but still manages to raise your heart rate to 50–70% of its maximum, which not only strengthens your heart but also burns serious calories. At a moderate walking pace you'll burn about five calories a minute, which means walking 20 minutes a day burns 100 calories a day (that's 8 lb (3.5 kg) of weight lost a year). And, by speeding up your metabolism, walking will continue to burn calories faster even when you're stationary.

And that's not all. Walking can significantly improve your mood (those endorphins again), with some scientists saying that a fast-paced walk can be even more effective than tranquillizers. Regular walking also helps stabilize your blood-sugar levels, helping to avoid mood and energy crashes, and boost your immunity. Stride out and you'll be strengthening the muscles in your hips, thighs, stomach, and bottom, while keeping osteoporosis at bay.

If you start walking to work, school, or evening social events (carry high heels in your bag), you'll not only save money on transport, but you'll also be able to fit into your life the recommended quota of 20–30 minutes or more of exercise five times a week. And practice a good walking technique. Walk tall with your stomach pulled in to support your back, and your shoulders relaxed and down so you can breathe more deeply. Wear sneakers or well-fitting flat shoes, and either swap your handbag from side to side or invest in a leather rucksack for even weight distribution.

How fast is fast enough? You should be able to talk, but if you can carry on an easy, effortless conversation then you need to pick up the pace. And don't forget to warm up and cool down (as you would with any exercise) by starting and finishing at a slower pace, plus be kind to your muscles with a few shoulder shrugs, arm swings, gentle forward bends, and hamstring stretches before and after your walk.

Find your rhythm

Anything that raises your heart rate and gets you breathing a little faster is good for your health (and stamina), which means dancing counts as exercise. It's the most sociable way to work out ever, or just turn up the music at home and discover your inner dancing queen. Don't underestimate the effect music has on your soul. The combination of music and movement has been proven to create high levels of energy, balance your heart rate, and release stress. Never felt confident on the dancefloor? Then take a class in flamenco, salsa, or belly dancing. Who said exercise was boring?

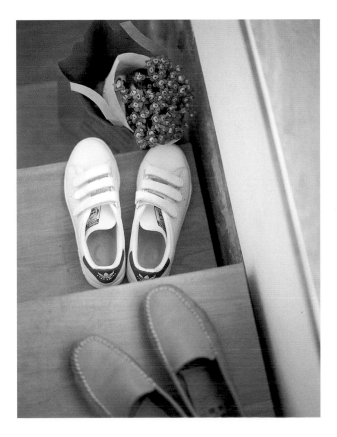

Child's Play: How to Have More Fun

When you are a child, exercise is all about having fun— running, skipping, and jumping until the school bell rings or bedtime beckons. But fast-forward 20 or more years and suddenly exercise has become a chore you know you should do, but somehow never quite feel like you want to.

The answer is to go back to child's play (with grown-up benefits). You can't do better than rebounding. Don't make the mistake of dismissing bouncing on a mini-trampoline as less serious than pounding the pavement jogging, or getting sweaty down at the gym. NASA has now incorporated rebounding into their astronaut training program, as they've found it to be 68% more efficient at increasing aerobic fitness than using a treadmill, plus it builds bone and muscle mass—

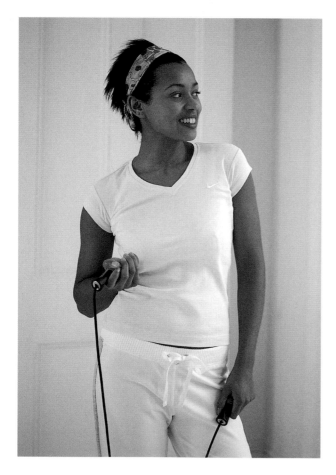

and helps combat osteoporosis. Just 10 minutes of bouncing is said to be the equivalent of half an hour's jogging, which also makes jumping up and down a very quick and efficient way to lose weight. And that's not all. Studies also show that bouncing on a mini-trampoline not only gives good cardiovascular benefits (without putting stress on your joints, making it perfect for anyone who is overweight or recovering from an injury), but also helps boost your lymphatic system by squeezing waste out of your cells. And by getting rid of toxins you'll be benefiting your skin and significantly reducing the appearance of cellulite. Do it daily for at least 5–10 minutes, to your favorite upbeat CD for best effects.

For more playful inspiration, think back to a time in your life when you were more physically active and loving it. You may have to go as far back as the school playground, or your teenage years. What did you enjoy most about it? The music, the fresh air, the people, the scenery? What are your memories of fun activities? A team sport like volleyball or basketball? Outdoor fun like rowing, horseback-riding, rollerblading, or cycling? Or learning an exhilarating new sport like skiing, diving, or ice skating? Think how you could do this again now. Some activities may be available nearby, or book an action-packed holiday to get you back in the mood.

If finding the time (or babysitter) to leave your house is a problem, you can now take classes with some of the world's finest fitness teachers in your own sitting room. There's a fitness DVD or video for everyone, from kickboxing to dissolve your anger (exercise has been proven to clear excess adrenaline), to aerobic dance so you can lose yourself in the music with no one looking.

The trick is to make it fun by not pushing your body too far, too fast. The more you do, the more your body will want to do, and the less you'll need to motivate yourself. If you need more inspiration, make a note of how you feel after your chosen activity and refer back to it should the sofa beckon. By making movement something you enjoy, it can easily become the highlight of your day rather than just another chore on your to-do list.

There's a fitness DVD or video for everyone, from **kickboxing** to dissolve your anger, to aerobic **dance** so you can lose yourself in the music with no one looking.

Beauty Sleep

From the number of hours spent in slumber to the way you lie on your pillow, how you sleep affects the way you age. Sleep is the cheapest and easiest anti-aging treatment available, and if you can fall asleep by 10 p.m. all the better, as the two hours before midnight are when your system (especially your stress glands) recharges and recovers. Deep sleep is what you're aiming for, as this is when cells are repaired and the human growth hormone (which slows aging) is released. Lack of sleep not only ages you, but is linked to health problems such as high blood pressure, a low immune system, and depression, not to mention making you irritable and unable to cope with what life throws at you (just ask any new mother).

Good-sleep strategies

* The darker your bedroom, the more melatonin you produce (a natural hormone which helps you fall asleep), so if your wooden blinds let in too much light, wear an eye mask (ear plugs are a godsend for noisy bedrooms, too). If you get up during the night, keep the main lights off, as a sudden flood of light switches off melatonin production.

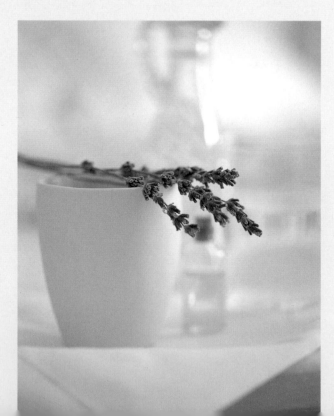

* The main cause of poor sleep is stress. If you've had a hard day, go for an evening walk to use up excess adrenaline.
* Avoid watching stimulating TV before bedtime and never read anything unrelaxing in bed. Remove televisions, laptops, and other distractions from your bedroom, too.
* Avoid caffeine (in coffee, tea, cola, and chocolate) and nicotine after 6 p.m., as they stimulate brain activity and raise blood pressure. The food additive MSG (commonly found in Chinese take-out and convenience foods) will have the same effect, as will very spicy food. And avoid eating a heavy, rich meal late at night—it may make you feel drowsy temporarily, but can seriously disrupt sleep by taking longer to digest, which wakes up your brain.
* Eat early in the evening, filling up on serotonin-rich foods (which also help increase melatonin production) like brown rice, whole-wheat pasta, couscous, and baked potatoes.
* Stop smoking, as nicotine is a stimulant and has been linked to problems falling asleep and waking in the night.
* Keep your feet warm with bedsocks or a hot-water bottle, as it's almost impossible to fall asleep with cold feet.
* If an uninterrupted night is but a distant memory due to young children, try taking 10-minute naps (but no longer) during the day, which will help do the job those eight hours did before.

Good-skin strategies

Lack of sleep can accelerate the aging process. Why? People deprived of good-quality sleep have higher levels of the stress hormone cortisol, which slows down the skin's natural repair functions.

* Dermatologists can usually tell which side you lie on by the "sleep wrinkles" on your face caused by pressing into the pillow. If you can sleep on your back, so much the better, but if not, slip a silk pillowcase over your cotton one to help reduce friction and pressure on your face.
* Traditional night creams are richer in texture than the average day cream, but you may prefer a more lightweight serum for night, which does the same job of hydrating the

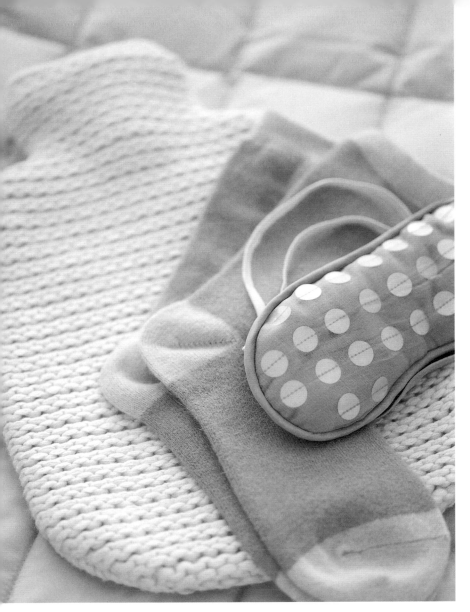

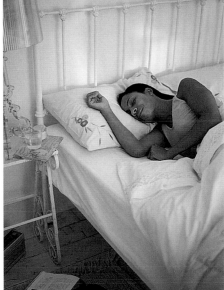

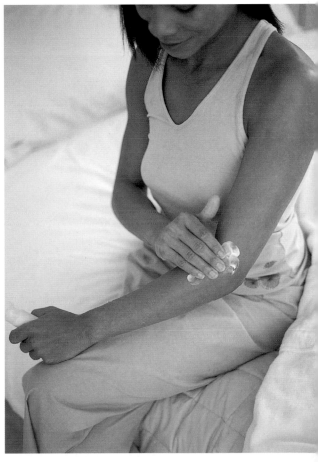

skin, without leaving it feeling greasy. Do you need a separate night product? Not really, but wearing a cream containing an SPF at night might overload sensitive skin with chemicals. Many skin experts advise leaving your face naked at night so it can "rebalance," which is worth a try if your skin has been misbehaving lately.

* Skin likes a well-ventilated, slightly humid room, so keep the central heating on low and keep air circulating through. Natural bedding such as linen, cotton, or silk will also allow skin to breathe—and feels much nicer, too.

* Establishing a mini bedtime wind-down ritual is the best way to allow your body and brain to leave the day behind. Brush your teeth and then apply your night-time moisturizer, gently moving your hands from the center of your face upwards and outwards while taking deep, abdominal breaths to release any tension in your body.

Ageless Energy   97

Keep a pad by your **bedside** so you can write down anything that's on your **mind** during the night and **deal** with it in the morning.

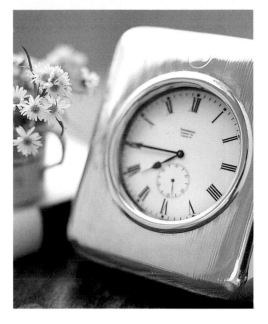

Solutions for Sleep Problems

3 If you do wake up in the night, never lie in bed for longer than 30 minutes. Go into another room and do something repetitive like unstacking the dishwasher, ironing, or knitting. You could also try eating tryptophan-rich food (like a small bowl of cereal with chopped banana), as this amino acid aids sleep. And put your alarm clock out of sight (under your bed or in your bedside cabinet), so you won't be tempted to lie in bed practicing your mental arithmetic ("If I don't nod off until 4 a.m. I'll only have another three hours until the alarm goes off at 7," and so on).

4 The time you wake up is as important for setting your body clock as the time you fall asleep, which means getting up at your regular time even if you were awake for a couple of hours in the night. Don't use the weekend to catch up on missed weekday sleep, or you'll be out of sync by Monday.

5 White noise (like the background sound of an air conditioner) can help induce sleep. Far more melodic is a relaxation CD of nature-based sounds such as rushing water, birdsong, or crashing waves. Play it low at night as you drift off, or have it ready to play should you wake up in the night.

6 You're more likely to feel sleepy when your body temperature drops after being warmed up, which is why a bath before bedtime can help you sleep (just don't make it too hot). Or try a hot foot bath, which helps calm the mind by diverting excess energy away from the brain. Soak your feet for 10 minutes or until the water cools.

7 Try not to worry about the sleep you have. When tested in laboratories, people who said they hardly slept at all actually got far more sleep than they thought, so if you're concerned about how many hours you're clocking up each night, keep a sleep diary of the times you drop off and wake up. You may be pleasantly surprised.

Every year, many people seek help for insomnia and sleep deprivation. If you're one of them, try these expert tips on how to nod off.

1 If you typically toss and turn in bed for at least an hour before falling asleep, you need to break the pattern your body clock has established. Do this by restricting the time you spend in bed and going to bed at least an hour later than normal. If you normally go to bed at 11 p.m. but don't fall asleep until 12:30, then put off going to bed until 12:30 and see what happens. It might just be a case of reconditioning yourself to sleep better simply by not going to bed until you feel like falling asleep.

2 Waking up a couple of hours after nodding off is often a sign of anxiety, so you need to look at what you're worrying about while you're conscious (rather than wait for your unconscious mind to nudge you awake in the night). Writing down what's on your mind literally works like a brain dump, getting the worry out of your head and onto paper, where you can devise a practical course of action. Make this a regular habit and niggling anxieties won't have time to grow and fester. Keep a pad by your bedside so you can write down anything that's on your mind during the night and deal with it in the morning.

The Many Joys of Sex

Sex is one of life's feel-good activities, and research says that women who have regular sex not only live longer but look at least 10 years younger, too. Pleasurable sex also releases hormones that help boost your immune system, reducing pain and stress levels. So why does sex sometimes seem like too much hard work? Just like exercise, rather than depleting your energy levels, regular sex improves your energy, and no one can fail to notice how radiant they look after an orgasm. In fact, orgasms don't just make you look and feel younger; they also relieve tension and produce phenetylamine, which helps reduce your appetite (the reason eating goes out of

the window when you're in the first stages of lust). Sex is also an invaluable part of bonding in a relationship, creating all those cosy feelings of love, security, and togetherness. An 80-year-old woman has the same potential for orgasm as a 20-year-old, so there's really no reason why sex should slip down your priority list as you get older.

Think yourself sexy

* Smell is a powerful stimulant, so never underestimate it. Wear a perfume you find sexy, or enhance your natural pheromones with essential oils like ylang ylang, musk, or vanilla. Sprinkle six drops in your bath or a few drops on your pillow or (sexy) nightgown.
* No one feels sexy in baggy sweatpants, so dress the part. Wear your best underwear, and clothes that make you feel good about yourself. And wear heels on a night out, for a sexy wiggle that's impossible in sneakers.
* Look after your body. So you may not look like those airbrushed models in the media, but nor do *they* in real life. Never fall into the trap of comparing yourself to these idealized images. Men don't, so why are you giving yourself such a hard time? Instead, make the most of what nature gave you with regular pampering sessions so your body always feels soft and smooth—a more attractive proposition to a man than any picture in a magazine.

Think him sexy

* Remember what you love and find attractive about your partner and, just as importantly, tell him. Men can have negative feelings about their bodies, too, so they need the same encouragement as you do.
* It's easy to get caught up in wanting your own way in a relationship, but life is much easier if you stop needing your partner to think the same as you in order to feel secure. And never is this more important than with sex. Don't automatically feel rejected if he's not in the mood. More beneficial is to recognize you both have different needs, and use your imagination to find a happy compromise.

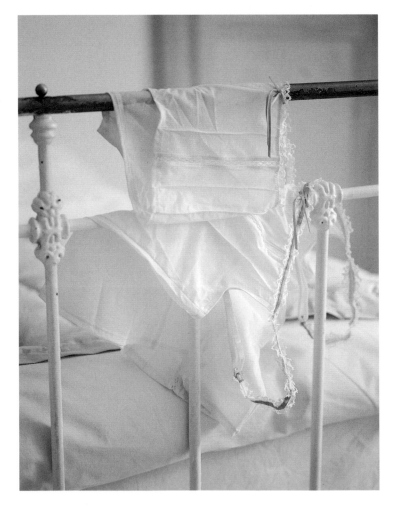

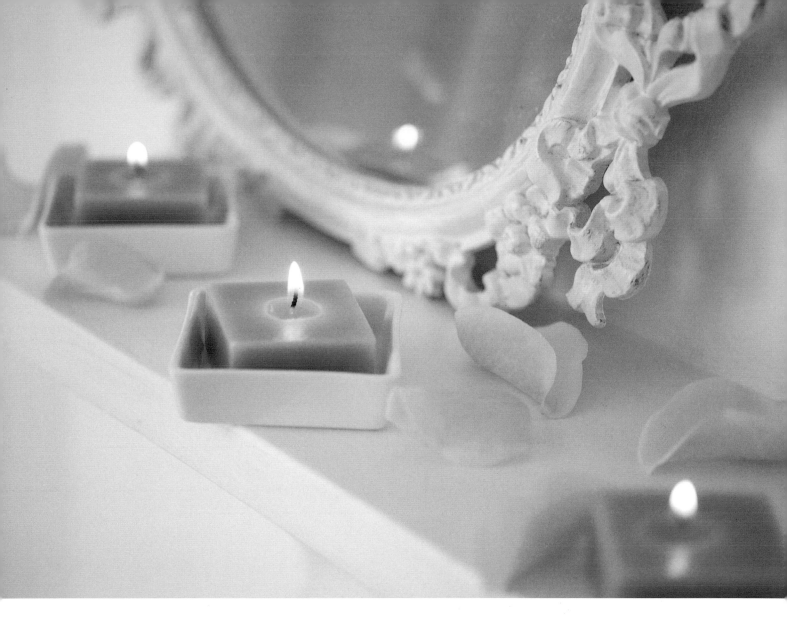

Boost both your libidos

* Sex and stress don't mix (stress lowers your level of testosterone, which controls your sex drive), so save sex for when there's time to enjoy it. Set the scene and the performance is bound to be more pleasurable. This might mean soft lighting, flowers, and a bubble bath, or romantic music and a candlelit dinner. Keep sex special and it won't lose its appeal.

* A poor diet will reduce the most rampant sex drive, so eat energy-boosting raw foods and cut down on stimulants such as sugar, coffee, cigarettes, and alcohol, which will exhaust you by the end of the day. High-fat and fast food is never going to make you feel sexy. Foods rich in zinc, like lean meat, nuts, eggs, and wholegrains, will, as zinc is very important for sexual function (oysters have a very high zinc content, too). Also important for the manufacture of sex hormones is vitamin E, so include plenty of wheat germ, dark green vegetables, avocados, almonds, and hazelnuts in your diet.

* If in doubt, start anyway. An active sex life triggers testosterone production, so the more you do it, the more you want to do it. Research says that many people with a low sex drive enjoy sex once they get started…

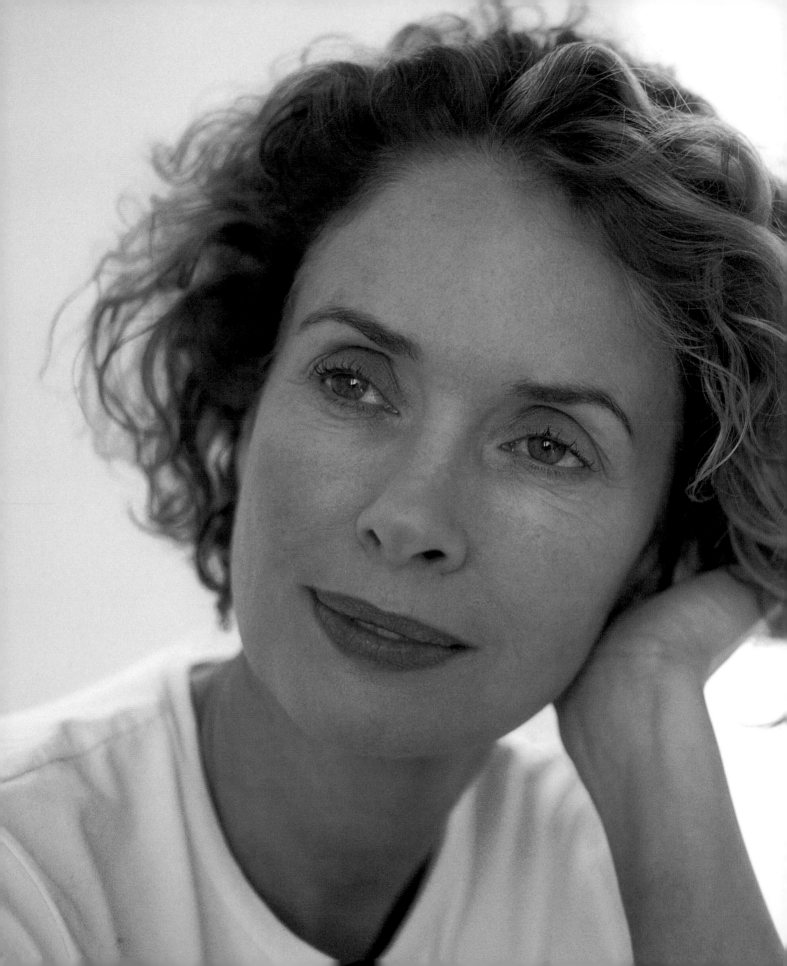

Ageless Mind
Keeping yourself powerfully positive

The Proven Power of your Mind

The single most important thing you can do to look and feel younger is to think positively about yourself. People who are more positive about life not only have a much happier one, but have also been found to live an average of eight years longer than their more pessimistic friends and family.

This comes as no surprise when you consider how important our thoughts are (see pages 82–83). Your body responds to what you tell it, which means that if you think you're youthful, desirable, or healthy, then your brain will look

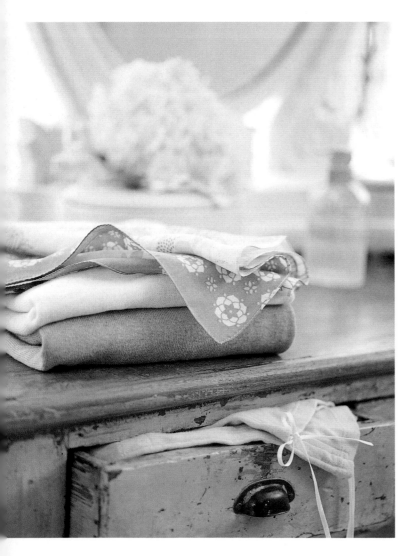

for evidence to support this. After all, it doesn't want to make a liar of you. The opposite is also true. If you constantly tell yourself that you're not as young as you used to be, your brain will prove it by finding examples of aging aches, pains, and wrinkles. But if you tell yourself you look and feel 10 years younger, your brain will show that to be true, too. Spoken affirmations may sound very "self-help," but you're doing them anyway, it's just that you're saying negative ones ("Look at the state of my bottom in this dress!"). So you may as well hijack them and switch to something far more supportive.

Retrain your brain

Your brain is like a computer, storing your interpretation of events on its hard drive. And that's the point. What you think becomes your reality, which means you can always reprogram your computer to start thinking younger. In one experiment, a group of people in their 70s and 80s were asked to think, behave, and dress as they had 20 years ago, and within five days their biomarkers (see pages 8–9) showed signs of age reversal.

Beliefs are extremely powerful. They are our explanations of how life is, and we collect them to help us get a sense of certainty in an unpredictable world. But we don't check whether they are still valid, and this means many are now no longer true (as a teenager, 40 probably really did seem ancient!). If you're not sure what you believe about your age, just notice how you look and feel every day. Are you stiff and sore first thing in the morning? Do you feel too old to exercise like you used to? Are your wrinkles the only thing you see in the mirror? Whatever you focus on, you'll experience more of, whether that's joint pain or sagging skin. Changing a belief can happen gradually (experts estimate it takes 21 days for a new habit to take hold), or as a flash of new insight (turn the page to find out how). Either way, be prepared to practice every day, as weakening old habits and building new ones is a little like muscle-strengthening exercises in the gym. It takes time and commitment, but the results are well worth it.

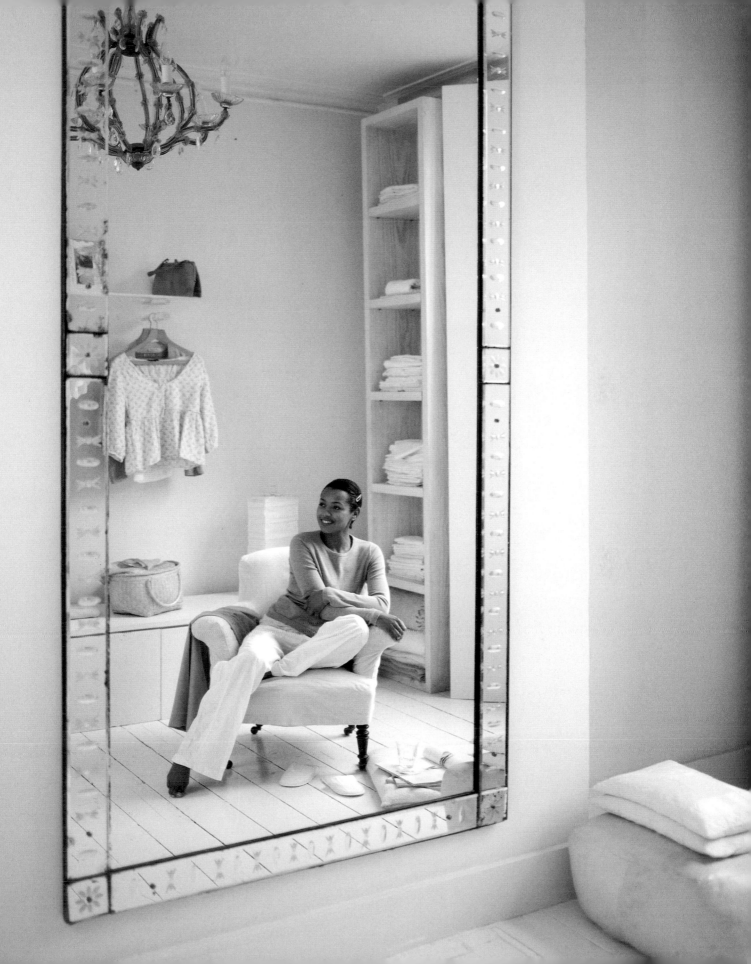

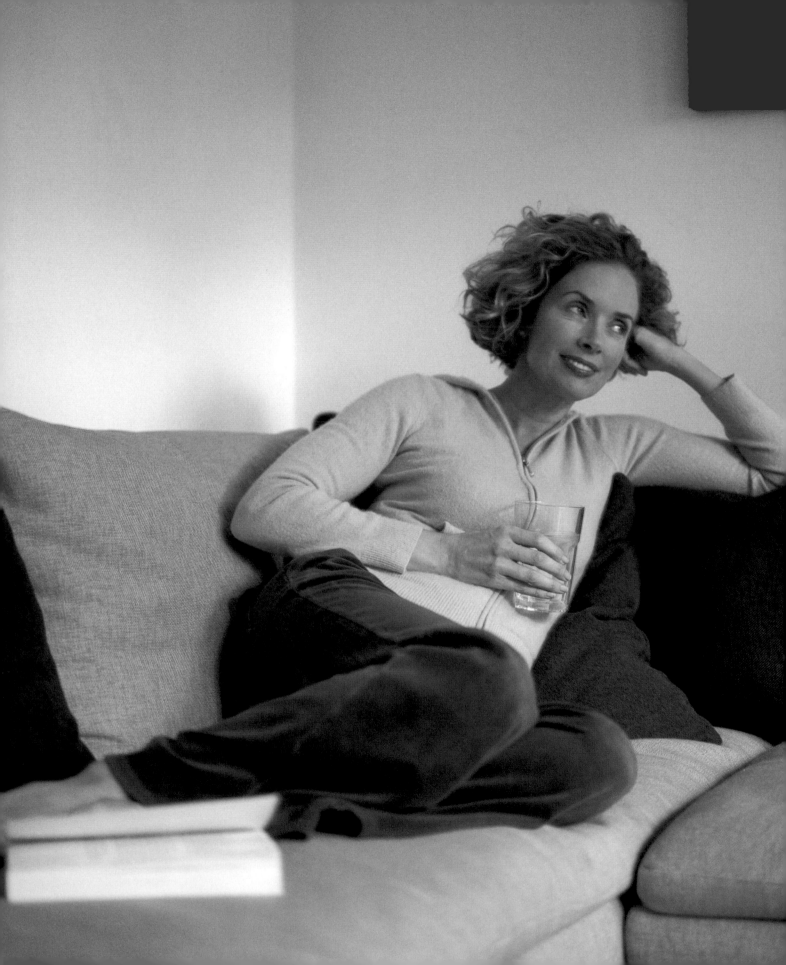

Anti-aging Mind Games

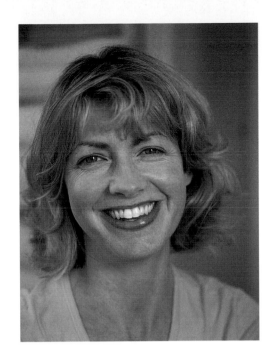

Change your beliefs

Is what you're saying to yourself useful? Remember that something is only the truth until new information comes along to contradict it. To change a belief, you must first identify exactly what it is that's working against you: "I'm too old to join a running club," "It's all downhill from here," etc. Then come up with a positive contradiction that will give you energy rather than drain you: "I'm 20 years younger than many marathon runners," "I feel better than I did five years ago." Write it down, repeat it at least five times a day, and start collecting evidence to support it. Even if your new belief is not completely true right now, keep thinking and acting as if it is. And, whenever you catch yourself focusing on what you no longer want to think, switch your focus by asking: What could be a more helpful way of looking at this?

Become an optimist

Think of an area of your life that you tend to be optimistic about (work, relationships, friends). What results do you usually get in this area? Now think of an area where you tend to be pessimistic. What results do you usually get in this area? The simple fact is this: if you tell yourself something is easy to do, it probably will be. Now you can see how you create your own results, choose something about yourself you would like to feel better about—your health, your fitness, your weight—and switch your attitude toward it. For the next month, whenever you think about this area, expect good things ("I'm never ill," "I'm getting fitter every day," "I look better in my clothes already"). When negative thoughts reappear, simply accept them and then quickly go back to your positive expectations. When you trust things will turn out well, they very often do.

Act the age you want to be

So, here's the challenge. Pick the age you want to be (it's most realistic to reduce your chronological age by anything up to 10 years), and then begin thinking that age. Say "I only feel…" five times a day. Dress more like you did then (unless your recent past includes boob tubes!), update your makeup (see pages 28–29), and ask your hairdresser to take 10 years off you (see pages 46–47). Rediscover your childhood self (see over) and do things you haven't done (or allowed yourself to do) for years. What did you love doing 10 years ago? Dancing? Going to festivals? Bowling? Camping? Running? Live your new age for at least a month, and see how you feel at the end.

Value yourself

A youthful body needs high-quality fuel, so eat as many anti-aging foods a day as possible, and avoid the ones that accelerate aging (see pages 64–67). If you find it difficult to treat your body with this level of respect, you need to take another look at your unconscious beliefs. Why do you believe you don't deserve the very best? Who are you still rebelling against? You now know how much your thoughts matter, so go back to "Change your beliefs" (above) and come up with a positive switch. "I value myself enough to only eat food that keeps me young and healthy" is a good start. Acting as if everything you do in your life matters really does make a lasting difference to what you're prepared to do (or are no longer prepared to do) to yourself.

Recapture your Youth

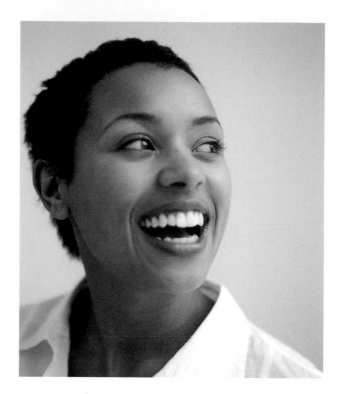

Remember how carefree you were as a child, with loads of fun and no responsibilities? You may be grown-up now, but that doesn't mean you can't stay young at heart.

Be spontaneous

As a child you did whatever came into your head that made you feel good. Now you have to plan three days ahead just to phone your best friend. Your week may feel like a never-ending to-do list, but that doesn't mean you can't find time to escape your diary. Unfortunately, the minute you plan something, it stops being spontaneous, so instead plan for nothing. Leave a day at the weekend completely free, and then when you wake up in the morning, ask yourself what exciting things you'll do today. The only rule is that they must make you feel good, just like when you were a child.

Play more

A playful adulthood (even more than a playful childhood) will boost your happiness levels, and more play in your life is now known to help you live longer, too. Play helps you test out situations, skills, and emotions without the consequences being too serious, which helps you in the real world as well. Play isn't passive (like sitting in front of the TV); it's energetic and creative. So don't just sit and watch as your (or a friend's) children play. Get in there and join in. Or play with your dog. Engage your friends in a game of charades. Or indulge in the ultimate adult play—brainstorming—at work or with friends and family. Keep the atmosphere relaxed and friendly, and encourage everyone to say whatever comes into their heads.

Be fearless

Remember when you dangled from that tree in the garden by one leg? Nowadays just putting the garbage out in the dark scares you. Children are born fearless, and they learn fear along the way. Some of this is good (those branches probably weren't that strong), but fear can stop you from doing so many things that would improve your happiness. If you're making excuses not to do something, look at what's behind your reaction. Chances are it's a fear of looking stupid, or failing, or being rejected, or just being out of your comfort zone. But this is the only way you achieve things in life. Ask yourself: What would I do if I wasn't afraid? Then work out the worst possible scenario. What if you didn't get that job you applied for? What if your date doesn't ask for another? If you can handle that, then you have nothing to fear.

Laugh more

Children laugh around 300 times a day, compared to adults, who manage a measly 17. But laughter is seriously good for you. It reduces stress hormones in your body, enhances immunity, releases toxins, relaxes muscle tension, and significantly improves your mood. Plus, an hour spent laughing could burn off as many as 300 calories. As children, we cry with laughter, but if you can't remember the last time you had a big belly laugh, you need to set it up to happen. When life's all too serious, you need something to switch your mood. So listen to a DJ who makes you laugh in the mornings, phone your funniest friend at lunchtime, visit a comedy club in the evening, or curl up on the sofa and watch a DVD of your favorite comedy show or stand-up comedian. A smile is the most inexpensive way to improve your looks, after all...

Leave a day at
the **weekend**
completely free,
and then when
you **wake up**
in the morning,
ask yourself what
exciting things
you'll do today.

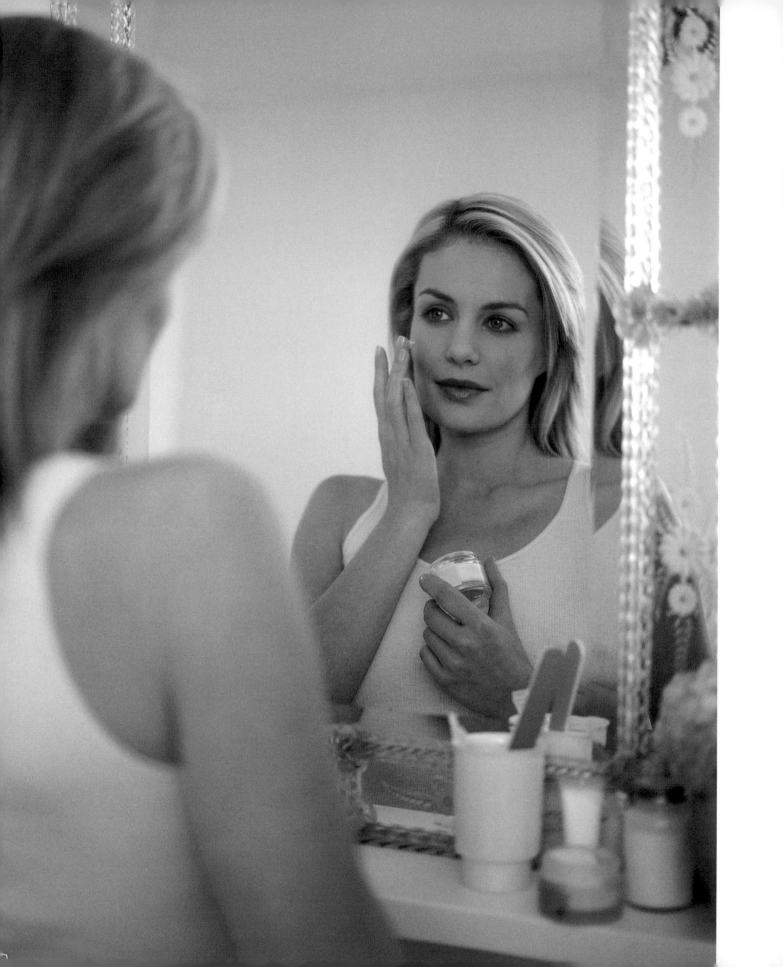

Living in the Moment

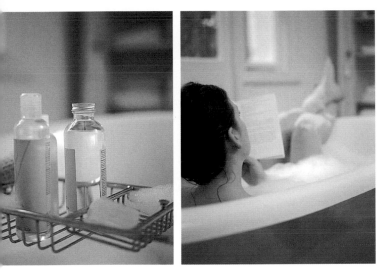

Spend your time in the past and nothing in the present will ever seem as good as it was then, not to mention making yourself feel ancient ("I remember back in 1982…"). Spend your time in the future and you'll just miss your life as it's happening. Children live in the moment, and regret nothing. Not so for adults, but you can't change the past and you certainly can't see into the future, so the best option is to take control of what's going on right under your nose.

Life is almost always fine in the present moment. Unless you're reading this standing in the path of an oncoming car, chances are everything's OK right where you are. So stop wasting energy on what you can't control, and instead concentrate on creating your life one day at a time to get the very best out of every single moment. Now is always the only time you can take action.

Decide to have a great day

This may sound simple, but you really do choose how you're going to feel every day. So if your intention is to have a good day, then that's probably what will happen. Do what it takes to start positive: play an upbeat CD while you're in the shower, eat your favorite breakfast, wear your best underwear, say "I love you" to yourself in the mirror (watch your feelings when you do this—it says a lot about how you feel about yourself!). And remember you can change your perspective at any moment, so if you find yourself assuming the worst about a situation, ask yourself: What else is possible? You may not be able to change the situation, but you can change your attitude towards it, and that's often all that's needed.

Give yourself something good to look forward to

Before getting out of bed, inspire yourself by deciding on your treats for the day. A walk in the park at lunchtime, lunch at your favorite cafe, a new magazine to read on the bus, a glass of wine in the bath before bed. Chances are the rest of your day will be taken up with tasks and chores for other people, so slipping in some stuff for yourself is well deserved. Make sure you do at least one thing that either feels great or produces great results (and preferably both) every day.

Fill your time with people and things you enjoy

Make a list of the most wonderful people you know and see or speak to at least one of them every day. Only eat food you really enjoy, and stop eating the minute you stop enjoying it. Read books and magazines you love (if you're bored by page 10, ditch it), and compile playlists of your favorite tunes. Life's too short to spend on things you don't enjoy (which might mean saying "no" a lot more often, too).

Expect good things to happen

We may not be able to create everything that happens in our lives, but we can certainly create how we view it. Our reality is really only our perception. The same day can happen to two people and they'll view it in a completely different way. One will see the problems, the other the fun and opportunities, and no prize for guessing who enjoys life more. Do you see the world as an unfriendly place? If so, take a day off from upsetting yourself and decide to see the best for a change. You never know, it might even happen.

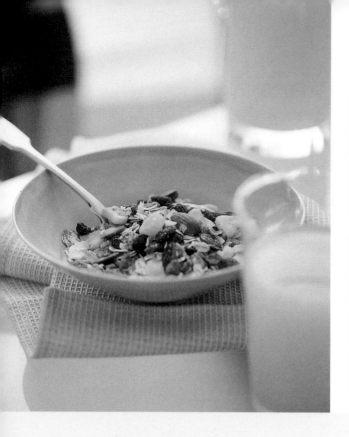
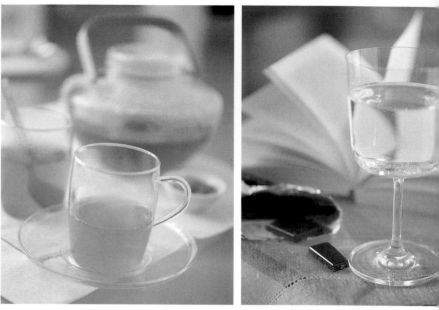

Long-life Habits

1 Get a morning kiss. Studies have found that people who enjoy a goodbye kiss are likely to live five years longer than those who leave the house without one.

2 Eat potassium-rich food every day. High-potassium foods such as bananas, raisins, and potatoes lower blood pressure, which significantly increases life expectancy.

3 Garden or spring-clean for five hours a week. Both activities burn on average five calories a minute, and studies have shown that people who burn 1,500 calories a week on gentle activities live 1.6 years longer than average.

4 Drink tea daily. Studies of heart-attack sufferers found their risk of having another in the next three years was cut by 44% if they drank two cups of antioxidant-rich tea a day.

5 Become a vegetarian. Whether it's due to less fat or more fruit, vegetables, and wholegrains in their diet, vegetarians live seven years longer than meat-eaters.

6 Eat a low-cholesterol diet. Studies say that people who live to 100 tend to have the lowest cholesterol, so cut down on your fat intake and eat carrots, apples, and avocados, which have all been shown to lower cholesterol levels.

7 Have at least six close friends or family members. People who don't have friends for support die up to 10 years earlier than more sociable souls.

8 Get a pet. Owning a pet helps you live longer, even when you've suffered a major illness. A study found that heart-attack sufferers increased their chances of being alive one year later by nearly five times if they owned a pet.

9 Drink alcohol in moderate amounts, but not in excess. Research has estimated that one or two alcoholic drinks a day (wine or beer) cut your risk of heart disease by 60%, but women who regularly drink more than their recommended 14 units a week die up to 10 years sooner than more moderate drinkers.

Studies have found that people who eat chocolate three times a week live five years longer than those who either don't eat any or eat more.

10 Learn to breathe more deeply. Studies have found that people who breathe deepest live longest, as deep breathing slows your heart rate and a slow heartbeat is associated with a longer life.

11 Eat a breakfast that includes wholegrain cereal or toast. Eating wholegrains cuts your risk of heart disease and cancer by 30%, adding an average of three years to your life.

12 Floss your teeth daily. According to US anti-aging expert Dr. Michael Roizen (see Directory), flossing your teeth reduces your risk of heart disease as the bacteria that cause gum disease also contribute to inflammation of the arteries.

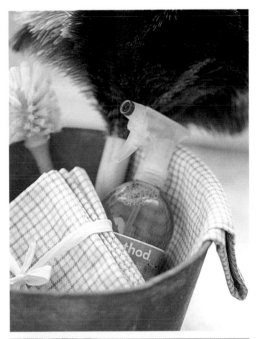

13 Eat chocolate in moderation. Studies have found that people who eat chocolate three times a week live five years longer than those who either don't eat any or eat more. This is probably due to chocolate's high antioxidant count, which is even higher than in fruit!

14 Stop smoking. It's estimated that every cigarette you smoke knocks 11 minutes off your life. And, according to pressure group A.S.H., women tend to smoke low-tar cigarettes, which makes them more prone to a particularly dangerous form of lung cancer.

15 Stay away from smokers. It's been estimated that a night spent in a smoky room is the equivalent of smoking four cigarettes yourself.

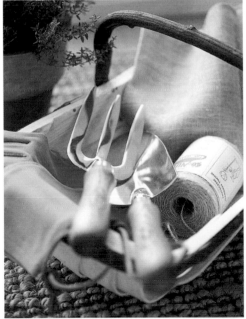

16 Go for regular health checks. This significantly increases your chance of surviving a major illness. Around 50% fewer women die of cervical cancer now that screening is widely available, and a mammogram can detect breast lumps two years before self-examination.

17 Stay a healthy weight. It's been calculated that every pound you're overweight knocks 36 days off your life. Studies have also found that eating significantly fewer calories (1,000–1,100 a day) can extend your life by up to 15 years.

How Stress Ages You

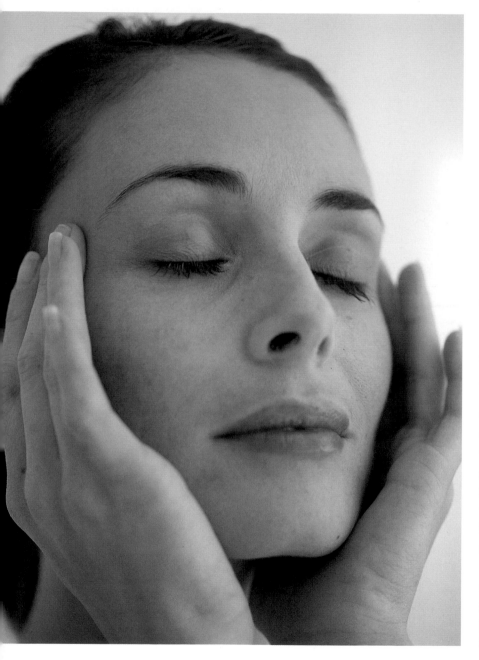

If you want to stay looking younger, you also need to stay calm. New research says psychological stress may be enough to age a woman's chromosomes by 10 years, as stress creates aging free radicals in your body. Our "fight or flight" response may have saved lives back when our ancestors needed to defend their territories, but nowadays it can kill.

If stress hormones have nowhere to go, they cause conditions such as high blood pressure, allergies, muscle tension, migraine, and headaches. And stress also worsens skin complaints like acne, rosacea (see pages 20–21), eczema, and psoriasis, all of which can increase skin aging. Stressful events can also cause hair thinning (see pages 48–49), although you may not relate the two, as hair fall normally starts around 10 weeks later. Stress can also turn you onto habits that accelerate aging, such as smoking, comfort eating, and excess alcohol.

The first signs of stress show up as tiredness, anger, or feeling unable to cope. Keep up that pace, and physical symptoms won't be far behind, including digestive problems such as irritable bowel syndrome, insomnia, and headaches. Stress hormones are also highly toxic and can trigger inflammatory conditions, including many of today's big killers: heart attacks, strokes, stomach ulcers, and cancer.

Stress can also be beneficial, helping you operate at your best, but you need to listen to your body and learn your limits. The moment you start to suffer, it's time to pull back and start some serious self-care.

Stress can help you **operate** at your best, but you need to **listen** to your body and learn your **limits**.

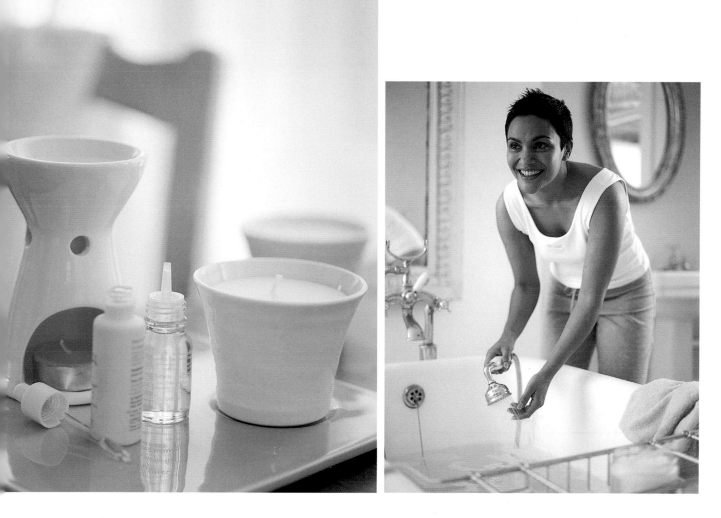

Dealing with stress

★ Don't underestimate how food can either help or hinder your ability to deal with stress. Stimulants will overwork your adrenal glands, making you even more jittery, so cut down your intake of caffeine, sugar, and alcohol. Anything that puts pressure on your digestion is also bad news, so steer clear of rich, heavy meals, refined and processed foods, and eating on the run.

★ Stress uses up the body's store of nutrients more quickly, so your first defense against it is a healthy diet. Add calming foods to your shopping list, such as whole-wheat pasta, oatmeal (the perfect breakfast before a stressful day), avocado, bananas, yogurt, turkey, and potatoes. Eat smaller meals regularly to balance your blood-sugar levels, and opt for easy-to-digest meals including smoothies, soups, and other sloppy foods.

★ Laughter releases stress (see page 108), as do getting eight hours of sleep a night (pages 96–99) and regular exercise sessions (pages 88–95). Learning how to slow down (see over) and meditate (page 85) will also work like first aid on frazzled nerves.

★ Complementary therapies such as aromatherapy massage, reflexology, acupuncture, flotation, and hypnotherapy can all work wonders on a mind under threat. And they'll help smooth frown lines, too.

★ Being conscious of exactly what causes you stress can go a long way to helping you cope with it. Keep a diary and write down when you're feeling most stressed. The aim is to respond rather than react, which may mean creating a space between what's stressing you and your reaction time. Take a walk, talk to someone you trust, or speak to a professional counselor or coach. An unbiased, outside perspective will help you see your situation more objectively, and when emotions are absent an intelligent solution is so much easier to find.

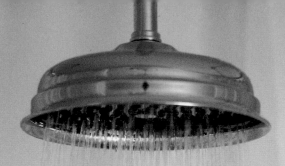

Often your **best** ideas come when you're doing something **mindless** and unrelated (on the train, in the bathtub), which is when your **unconscious** mind can nudge its way forward.

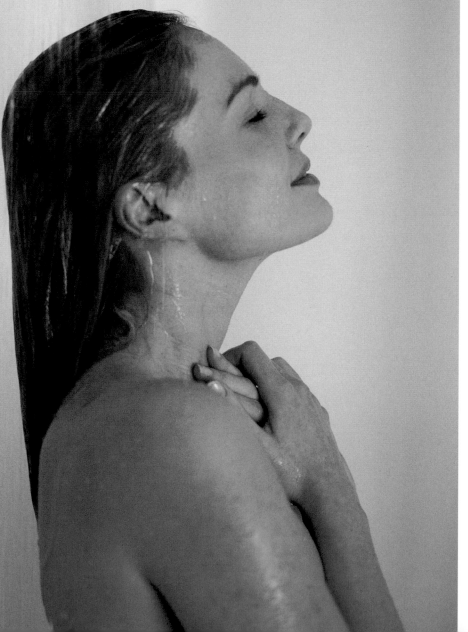

Slow Down (and be More Efficient)

The faster you go through life, the sooner the game is over. Just because everyone else is rushing doesn't mean you have to. Slow down, and you might find you achieve more, too.

Listen for longer

In today's high-speed society it's tempting to interrupt and make snap decisions to save time. Neither of these will make the other person feel heard. Letting them have their say will give you more information so you can then make a better decision, plus the other person is more likely to be more positive towards your suggestions in the future. Learn to listen three times better than you do now and you'll be amazed how well others respond.

Listen to your truth

Feeling the need to come up with an answer immediately is a massive pressure, so get comfortable with not always knowing right away. After all, why should you? Being confident enough to say "I don't know" is very attractive. Then you can go away and research the right answer rather than having to stick with the first thing that springs to mind. And the same thing applies the next time someone asks for a favor—pause and think what feels right for you before you say yes.

Listen to your (and others') mistakes

At the end of each day, take time to reflect on what you've learned. Making mistakes simply means you can do a task better next time, with more skill and in less time. And don't just learn from your own mistakes. The most successful people have learned by watching others—at a fraction of the cost.

Listen to your unconscious

If you tend to react fast, invent a buffer such as "That's interesting, let me think it over," and then allow yourself time to do just that. Often your best ideas come when you're doing something mindless and unrelated (on the train, in the bathtub), which is when your unconscious mind can nudge its way forward. Or get in touch with your intuition by softening your gaze into peripheral vision mode. Deferring judgment often leads to a better, faster solution in the end.

Listen to your thoughts

It's important to allow yourself a break and simply watch your mind do its thing without trying to control the pace. This helps you detach yourself from the millions of thoughts you have each day, so you can see what's valid and what's not. Give yourself at least 15 minutes a day to sit and do absolutely nothing but watch your thoughts go by. It's not only deeply relaxing, but can be very productive, too (see above). If your internal dialog threatens to overwhelm, simply close your eyes and make a "ssshhh" sound as though you're trying to lull a baby back to sleep. It will have the same quieting effect on your chattering brain.

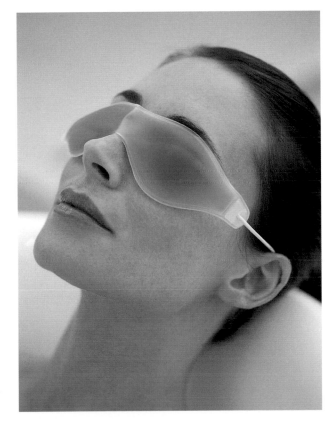

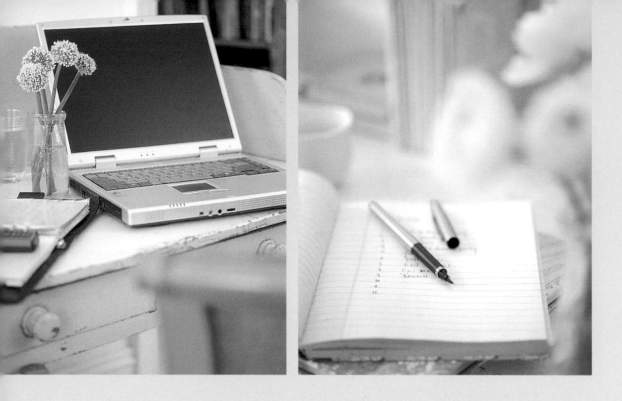

Give yourself More Time (in Every Sense)

We all have the same hours in a day we've always had, so why are we so busy? New technology saves us time, but we simply use what time we gain to cram more work in. The consequences of constantly racing against the clock include everything from skin and digestive problems to an early grave. If your time is flying, here's how to be the pilot.

Get up early

The simplest way to gain more time! Set the alarm half an hour earlier and see how much less frantic mornings can be.

Start as you mean to go on

Ditch the headless chicken act and *think* before you start the day. It's so easy to get caught up doing the wrong things, but if you're clear about your priorities before you begin, then you may end up doing less—but you'll do the right things. The most important choice we can make in our lives is what we choose to make important. What are your biggest priorities? Write them down and refuse to get sidetracked until they are successfully completed. Scared you'll forget the rest? They can go on your "some other day" list.

Make new technology work for you

Take the time to learn how to use new technology and exploit what it can do. Internet shopping and banking save you from standing in long lines, paying bills and managing accounts online saves you from call-center hell, and text messages save you from getting tied up in a long conversation when you've got other things to do.

Be ready for a time windfall

If you do get stuck in a long line, think of it as "found time." Practice what you're going to say in tomorrow's meeting, or to a difficult relative. Make the most of travel time by writing letters on the train or catching up on (hands-free) phone calls in a traffic jam. Carry a notebook with you so when you're hanging around with nothing to do, you can plan your next dinner party or simply ponder your life. Nothing takes the busy-ness out of your brain faster than writing down your thoughts. Why? Everything looks so much more manageable on paper. Or just daydream—it's good for your health.

Relaxing is not the same as collapsing—
it's simply time to switch off and regain your
sanity. If you can't see another way, ask a
friend who may see things **differently**.

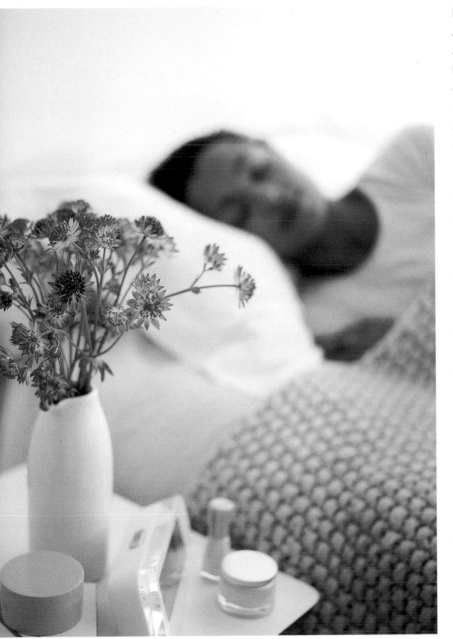

Know what works best for you

Are you a morning person who can accomplish a full day's work by lunchtime? Then get your head down first thing and ask colleagues not to disturb you. Do you come to life in the evening? If so, don't stress about your natural slow start, and know that you can catch up later when the early birds are falling asleep on the sofa.

Don't be a slave to your schedule

You control your time, not the other way around. How many hours this week have you spent on "empty" activities—TV? Complaining? What could you cut back on? Only watch programs you're really interested in? Focus on the good stuff in your life rather than moaning about the rest? And what about how other people misuse your time—listening to friends' problems, running errands for family members? What can you delegate or outsource? When do you need to say no? This little word is the greatest time-saver ever invented, and is totally justified when what you're being asked to do is less important to you than what you'd already planned.

Change your perspective

Are you really overwhelmed, or do you secretly enjoying playing the martyr? Today's "more is better" culture tells us that doing nothing is lazy, so we cram our lives full of activity. But relaxing is not the same as collapsing—it's simply time to switch off and regain your sanity. If you can't see another way, ask a friend or professional who may be able to see things differently.

Last Word: The Good News About Getting Older

There's never been a better time to get old. For centuries being old meant poverty and worse (menopausal women in the 17th century were said to cause grass to dry up and trees to die!). Pensions are barely 100 years old, and ones you can live on are even more recent. But if it's the best time in history to be old, why are we all so worried about it?

How happy we feel about each birthday depends very much on the beliefs we have about getting older. Do you see it as all downhill from here on? Do you believe your best years have already happened? If so, you'd better develop a more positive attitude toward aging, because it's going to happen to you—if you're lucky.

Are you frightened of getting older?
Take the fear of aging away with some preventative work. What are you doing now (a healthy diet, exercise, savings) to ensure yourself a great future?

How are you using your age as an excuse?
What are you not doing for fear of looking foolish or failing (going back to college, learning to snowboard, taking a long-overdue year off)? What would you do if you decided to admit your fear, but do what you feared anyway?

Do you cling to cherished memories of your "glory years"?
If so, list all the ways in which your life is better now than it was 10 years ago.

Does the exciting part of your life seem over?
Then take time to list all the things you'd like to do in the next 10 years and start to get at least three projects up and running as soon as possible.

Chances are it's not time you're afraid of, but change. Accept that nothing lasts forever and you'll find it far easier to enjoy what's going on at any age. You may have had firmer thighs 10 years ago, but you were probably too busy obsessing about something else you didn't like, to find time to appreciate them. So stop focusing on getting older, and concentrate on getting wiser. There was a time when we believed the brain decayed with age, but research now says that staying mentally active causes the brain to sprout new connections between nerve cells. This means you create your brain from the input you get—plus "growing" your brain by learning new things all your life is the best way to avoid diseases such as Alzheimer's and strokes.

The truth is, most of us feel more at home with ourselves as we get older. You have made yourself who you are and, if life's good, that's better than being any angst-ridden youth. And if it's not, now's the time to get smarter. It's easy to gain wisdom as you age if you consider your part in why events happened in your life and learn from those experiences. Age also gives you the confidence to see your priorities more clearly and do exactly what you want. If not, what are you saving your best self for? The older you get, the healthier you've been, which in itself is a cause to celebrate. Perhaps it's time to grow young at 40 (or 50). Your lips may be slightly thinner, but your smile can be twice as wide.

Fear less, hope more
Whine less, breathe more
Talk less, say more
Hate less, love more
And all good things are yours.

SWEDISH PROVERB

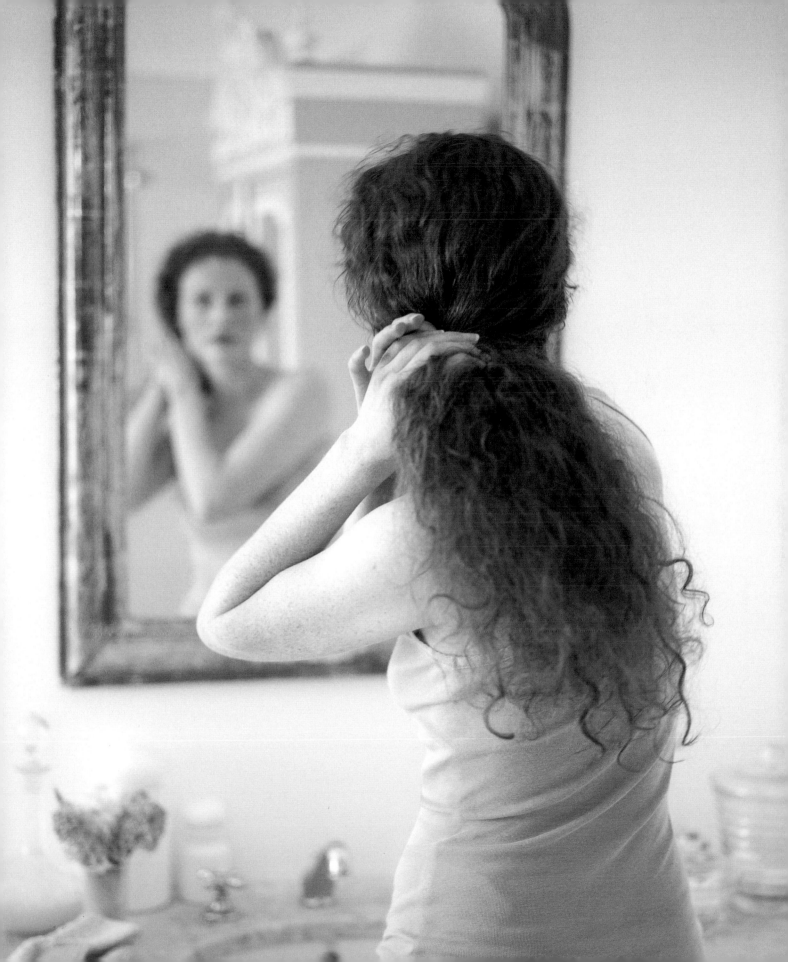

Directory

Skincare, natural makeup, and toiletries organizations

American Academy of Anti-Aging Medicine
888-528-4333, www.worldhealth.net
Directories of clinics and products, anti-aging tips and publications.

American Academy of Dermatology
P.O. Box 4014
930 North Meachum Road
Schaumburg, IL 60168
847-330-0230, www.aad.org
To find a board-certified dermatologist.

www.rosacea.org
1-888-NO-BLUSH
Describes symptoms, treatments, and trigger factors.

The Skin of Color Society
1-800-460-9562
www.skinofcolorsociety.org
To find a dermatologist specializing in skin of color.

Skincare products

Clinical Creations, LLC
1-888-823-7837
www.clinicalcreations.com
Learn what causes wrinkles and beauty treatments, nutritional tips, and supplements to combat them.

For information about Daniel Sandler, visit www.danielsandler.com.

Dermalogica
310-900-4000, www.dermalogica.com
Visit the website to locate a skincare therapist trained by The International Dermal Institute (www.dermalinstitute. com) and where to buy Dermalogica, which may be purchased only from salons.

Liberty Natural Products
1-800-289-8427
www.libertynatural.com
Natural healthcare products, aromatherapy, and natural perfumes.

Lush
www.lush.com
Fresh handmade cosmetics.

Jane Iredale Mineral Makeup
www.janeiredale.com

Natural Web Store
1-800-830-5877
www.naturalwebstore.com
Natural beauty care products, vitamins and herbal supplements, and more.

Sephora
1-877-SEPHORA, www.sephora.com
Designer cosmetics and skincare.

Shop Natural
www.shopnatural.com
Natural health and beauty aids.

Skin Biology, Inc.
1-800-405-1912, www.skinbiology.com
Products include mineral sunscreens.

The Susan Ciminelli Day Spa
www.susanciminelli.com
Anti-aging products and information.

Cosmetic surgery

American Society for Aesthetic Plastic Surgery
888-272-7711, www.surgery.org
Information on cosmetic surgery; referrals.

American Society of Plastic and Reconstructive Surgeons
444 East Algonquin Road
Arlington Heights, IL 60005
847-228-9900, www.plasticsurgery.com
To find a board-certified surgeon.

The Center for Dermatology, Cosmetic, and Laser Surgery
359 East Main Street, Mount Kisco, NY
914-241-30
www.thecenterforderm.com
Resource for dermatology, cosmetic procedures, and skincare products.

Botox and other treatments

BotoxCosmetic.com
1-800-433-8871 (Allergan, Inc.)
Website explains the whys and hows of Botox treatments; doctor referrals.

Folica
1-888-919-4247, www.folica.com
Home microdermabrasion treatments.

See also Cosmetic Surgery for organizations that provide referrals for these cosmetic procedures.

Teeth

Academy of General Dentistry
211 East Chicago Avenue, Suite 900
Chicago, IL 60611
888-AGD-DENT, www.agd.org
Reliable dental health information.

American Academy of Cosmetic Dentistry
800-543-9220, www.aacd.com

GoSmile
110 East 42nd Street, Suite 1301
New York, NY 10017
877-8-SMILES
Visit gosmile.com for information on this home-whitening system.

Tom's of Maine
www.tomsofmaine.com
Socially responsible toothpaste and other personal-care products made from natural ingredients. Available at your local drugstore.

Eyelash extensions

Lavish Lashes
1-877-433-1790
www.lavishlashes.com
Contact to locate a local professional certified in applying extensions.

Xtreme Lashes
1-877-BIG-LASH
www.xtremelashes.com
Contact to locate a certified professional.

Nails
Hooked on Nails
www.hooked-on-nails.com
Natural nail care.

Jessica Vartoughian
1-800-582-4000
www.jessicacosmetics.com

Natural Market
1-800-439-5506
www.naturalmarket.com
Natural nail-care products.

Hair
Aveda
www.aveda.com
Herbal hair-care products and salons.

Glenn Lyons, at Philip Kingsley
+44 20 7629 4004

HairColorist.com
Directory of colorists in your area.

Herbatint Permanent Herbal Hair Color
is available at www.iHerb.com or call
1-888-328-1171 (Papanature).

International Association of Trichologists
(North American office)
Kalamazoo, MI
616-372-3224

Paul Matthews
+44 20 7240 1113

Steven Goldsworthy
+44 1793 523817

Skin nourishing supplements
Bronson Pharmaceuticals
4526 Rinetti Lane
La Canada, CA 91011
1-800-521-3322
High-quality vitamins and minerals.

See also Clinical Creations (under
Skincare Products).

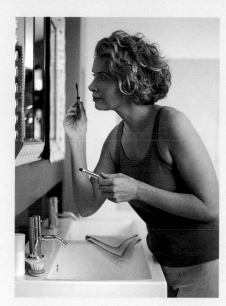

Life Extension Foundation
P.O. Box 229120
Hollywood, FL 33022
800-544-4400 (orders)
www.lifeextensionfoundation.org
Nonprofit dedicated to anti-aging; good
source for hard-to-find supplements.

Optimum Health
1-800-228-1507, www.opthealth.com
Exclusive selection of health-care
supplements for total body wellness.

Udo's Choice Oil is available at health
stores nationwide and through the online
sources listed in this section.

The Vitamin Shoppe
1-800-223-1216, www.vitaminshoppe.com
Vitamins and herbal supplements.

General medical information
American Cancer Society
800-ACS-2345, www.cancer.org
Info about smoking cessation programs,
skin cancer, and other resources.

National Institute of Health
www.nih.gov
Health information and consumer health
publications on many topics.

U.S. Food and Drug Administration
www.fda.gov
Check for cosmetics-related issues and
the latest results of FDA safety testing.

Energy
Feldenkrais Educational Foundation
of North America
1-866-333-6248, www.feldenkrais.com
Find a certified practitioner.

Pilates Method Alliance
1-866-573-4945, www.pilatesmethod.org
Resources and referrals from the only
accredited Pilates designation in the U.S.

Transcendental Meditation
1-888-LearnTM, www.tm.org

T'ai Chi
www.scheele.org/lee/tcclinks.html
Extensive list of websites offering
information about t'ai chi and
teacher referrals.

Yoga Finder
www.yogafinder.com
Links to yoga teachers, workshops,
and retreats.

Inner age tests
HB Health, www.hbhealth.com.

The RealAge Test, www.realage.com
Oprah-endorsed inner age test.

Useful books and information
Eva Fraser's Facial Workout is available at
bookstores, or visit www.evafraser.com
for DVDs and online courses.

Real Age: Are You as Young as You Can Be?
by Dr. Michael Roizen is available at
bookstores and Amazon.com.

Liz Wilde
Visit www.wildelifecoaching.com for
information about Liz Wilde's online
programs and one-to-one coaching.

Index

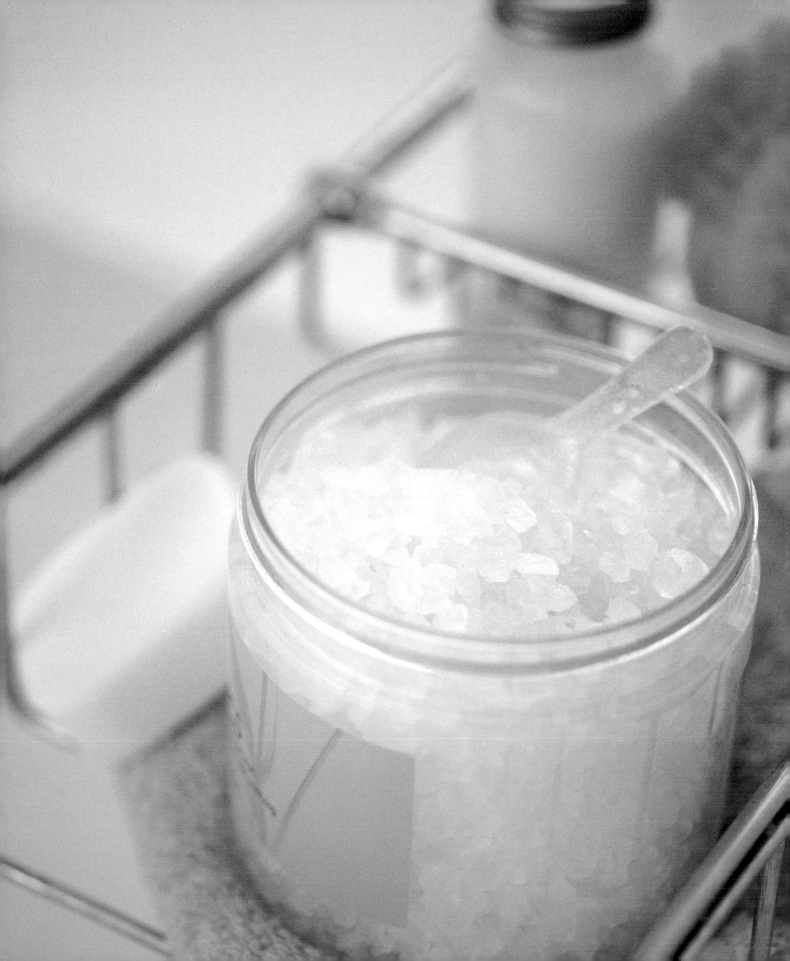

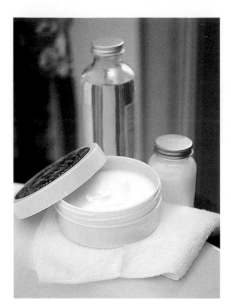

Picture Credits

All photography by Winfried Heinze unless otherwise stated.

Key: ph=photographer, a=above, b=below, r=right, l=left, c=center

Pages 8–9 ph Debi Treloar; 63r ph David Montgomery; 65r ph Dan Duchars; 66l ph Debi Treloar; 66r ph Ian Wallace; 75b ph Dan Duchars; 80c ph Peter Cassidy; 80r ph Debi Treloar; 81b ph Dan Duchars; 82 & 92 ph Polly Wreford; 99 ph Dan Duchars.

Acknowledgments

The publishers would like to say thank you to all our lovely models, especially Emily, Kathy, Jayne, Jacqui, Kelly, Carol Ann, Zena, Amanda, Melanie, and Anna.

Very special thanks also to Kelly at Allsorts, Kate at MOT Models, and Sally at Norrie Carr Agency.

With thanks to R. K. Alliston for the loan of props for photography.
R. K. Alliston
173 New King's Road
London SW6 4SW
+44 845 1305577
www.rkalliston.co.uk